Mastering Health

The A to Z of Chi Kung

Chi is the universal
energy that fuels
both the physical and spiritual universe.
Fill yourself with this vibrant energy, through the
ancient method of Chi Kung,
and meet any challenge with dynamic physical
power and positive mental focus.

MASTERING HEALTH

THE A TO Z OF CHI KUNG

SCOTT SHAW

New Age Books

ISBN: 81-7822-272-8

First Indian Edition: Delhi, **2006**

Reprinted from *Chi Kung for Beginners*
published 2004, by Llewellyn Publications
St. Paul, MN 55164, U.S.A.
www.llewellyn.com

Interior photos courtesy of Scott Shaw

Disclaimer

The practices, techniques, and meditations described in this book should not be used as an alternative to professional medical treatment. This book does not attempt to give any medical diagnosis, treatment, prescription, or suggestion for medication in relation to any human disease, pain, injury, deformity, or physical condition. The author and publisher of this book are not responsible in any manner whatsoever for any injury which may occur through following the instructions contained herein. It is recommended that before beginning any alternative healing practice you consult with your physician to determine whether you are medically, physically, and mentally fit to undertake the practice.

Published by
NEW AGE BOOKS
A-44 Naraina, Phase I
New Delhi-110 028 (INDIA)
Email: nab@vsnl.in
Website: www.newagebooksindia.com

For Sale in Indian Subcontinent Only

Printed in India
at Shri Jainendra Press
A-45 Naraina Phase-I, New Delhi-110 028

Contents

Contents

Introduction

Modern science teaches us that every element of this universe, from the smallest subatomic particles to the largest planet, is pulsating with energy. Over two-thousand years ago, in ancient China, this energy was defined as *Chi.*

In the modern era, Chi is commonly understood to mean "Internal Energy." Chi is much more than that, however. Chi is the universal energy that gives rise to all elements of life and fuels both the physical and spiritual universe. Chi cannot be seen; it cannot be touched. Yet, those who have interacted with this universal energy can attest to the fact that it does, in fact, exist.

Because Chi is such an abstract science, many people believe that the ability to consciously access this energy is only available to monks who live in caves or advanced martial artists who practice esoteric styles of *Kung Fu.* This is not the case. The energy of Chi can be brought into the life of any individual who wishes to perform a few simple exercises.

From the third century BCE forward, it has been understood that the human breath is what links the individual to the cosmic energy of Chi. From this knowledge, there have been very exacting techniques developed that instruct a person to effectively harness this power. These exercises are known by the Chinese term, *Chi Kung.*

The primary method to consciously bring the energy of Chi into the human body is through advanced methods of breath control. This science is based in the understanding that we, as human beings, are elementally dominated by breathing. We can live several days without food, a few without water, but the moment we are robbed of our breath, life as we know it ceases to exist.

With this imperative connection to breath as a basis of understanding, the ancient founders of Chi Kung acutely refined the methods for the intake of breath, whereby the practitioner could come to a higher and more profound level of human interaction with the universal energy of Chi.

In this book, the ancient method of Chi Kung will be detailed. With practice, you will possess the ability to consciously become interactive with this universal energy, and be able to tap into it in times of physical or mental need. By becoming consciously interactive with Chi you will be able to instantly summon up enhanced, and seemingly supernatural, amounts of physical and mental energy. No longer will you feel rundown, lackadaisical, or spiritless. Instead, you will be filled with the vibrant source of energy that fuels this universe, and you will be able to meet any challenge with dynamic physical power and positive mental focus.

chapter one

Chi Kung Preparation

Chi is a science that has been practiced and handed down for centuries. Similar to the music that comes from the speakers of your stereo, Chi cannot be seen but can be experienced. As Chi cannot be physically seen or touched by the untrained individual, there are many who do not believe in the power of this ancient understanding.

Chi is a mental science. As such, to begin to experience its power, you must initially possess at least a general belief in this understanding. From this step of faith, once you begin the practices of Chi Kung detailed in this book you will quickly begin to encounter the power of this ancient knowledge.

Preparing to Touch Chi

Though Chi is universally available, most people do not understand how to readily access this energy. Therefore, throughout the centuries there have been exacting methods devised to bring you into contact with this energy in the most expedient fashion possible.

To begin your practice of Chi Kung there are a few preliminary understandings you must possess. By employing these techniques you will begin to come into conscious contact with Chi. Thus you will bypass many of the obstacles that have the potential to keep you from rapidly becoming empowered with this universal energy.

Chi and Your Breath

You can live a few days without water, several days without food, but you can only exist for a few moments without air. The air you breathe is the most vital key to your life.

You can expand upon this basis of knowledge by looking to modern medical science and viewing statistics that prove the individual who is actively involved in cardiovascular activities is the least prone to many types of physical and mental ailments. Thus, from a strictly scientific point of view, those who take in the most oxygen are the most healthy.

The Chi Kung practitioner actively brings in excess amounts of oxygen into the body, not solely from an athletic vantage point, but from very refined methods of breath control. Thus the ancient science of Chi Kung teaches what modern medicine has, only in the recent past, begin to understand—oxygen is good.

Chi Kung teaches that Chi is consciously brought into your body via your breath. The Chi Kung practitioner comes to understand that no longer is breathing simply an unconscious act. Instead, it is embraced as a pathway to not only enhanced physical and mental well-being but a way to come into contact with the divine energy of this universe as well.

The Two Breaths of Chi

There are two distinct techniques of breathing directly associated with Chi Kung, *Zhen Hu Zi,* "Normal Breathing," and *Fan Hu Zi,* "Reverse Breathing."

Normal breathing is the natural pattern of breathing. When you breathe in, your chest and stomach expand. This style of breathing, when used in association with Chi Kung, is also known as "Buddha Breathing," as this was the style of breathing used by ancient Buddhist practitioners of Chi Kung.

Reverse Breathing is the process of reversing this natural process—when a breath comes in, your chest and stomach contract. This style of breathing, also known as "Taoist Breathing," was the breathing style that ancient Taoist practitioners of Chi Kung put to use.

Proponents of each style of Chi Kung breathing will argue their case as to the superiority of one method over the other. If we look at nature, however, we see that a baby's chest naturally expands when they breathe in. With this as our guide, it is suggested that you breathe in the natural pattern when practicing the Chi Kung techniques presented in this book. You should allow the natural process to ultimately be your guide in relation to Internal Energy.

The Two Types of Chi

There are two distinct types of Chi that are linked to the practices of Chi Kung. The first is known as *Wai Chi,* or "Outer Chi," and the second is *Nei Chi,* or "Internal Chi."

Wai Chi is the Chi that empowers the universe around you. This is the Chi that you consciously take in through your breath when you perform Chi Kung. Wai Chi is the element of Chi that provides you with a new and unlimited source of energy.

Nei Chi, or Internal Chi, is the energy that you consciously unleash into your body, from your central energy point. The techniques associated with this process will be discussed in the following pages.

The Two Types of Chi Kung

There are two specific styles of Chi Kung. They are *Tung Kung,* "Active," and *Ching Kung,* "Passive."

Active Chi Kung represents the methods of breath control from a position either standing, seated, or lying down. These are the exercises that directly cause Chi to rapidly come into and effectively circulate throughout your body.

Passive Chi Kung, on the other hand, is utilized by the practitioner who, through years of practice, has transcended the need for additional amounts of Chi to nourish their internal or external beings. This occurs when you have purified your body to the degree that Chi has permeated your being. Thus, you are constantly interactive and, in fact, a direct channel for this cosmic energy. At this point your only focus is upon that of meditation.

Sitting

When you perform seated Chi Kung, it is advisable that you sit in the cross-legged Lotus Posture. This posture naturally "locks" Chi energy into your upper torso. As several Meridians end in your legs or feet, Chi energy, that has been consciously brought into your body, has the potential to escape unnoticed through these bodily elements.

As seated Chi Kung techniques were designed to be practiced in this fashion for highly refined reasons, unnatural loss of Chi will cause your Chi Kung exercise to provide less-than-adequate results. The Lotus Posture naturally keeps this from occurring.

Due to age, arthritis, or previous injuries, many people have trouble sitting in this position. If this is your situation, there are two things you can do. One, slowly develop the ability to sit in this posture during short periods of practice. When you are doing this you should not attempt to perform Chi Kung because the discomfort you are experiencing will distract you from the actual technique, and your results will be substantially minimized. Simply sit and make yourself comfortable with this posture.

The second thing you can do is to sit in a chair, with your spine erect. The best way to keep your body consciousness while performing Chi Kung from this position is to sit several inches away from the back of the chair. Sitting in this fashion, you will not become too relaxed.

If you perform seated Chi Kung in this manner, you must remain very conscious about the possibility of escaping Chi particularly through your feet. Therefore, it is important to wrap a blanket or towel around your feet if you practice seated Chi Kung, no matter what temperature it is outside. With your feet naturally warmed, Chi energy will not naturally flow to that region of your body to warm it. You will then be saved from unnecessary Chi loss.

Standing

Many Chi Kung exercises are performed from a stationary standing position. As all Chi Kung practices are performed with interactive mental consciousness as the elementary focus, so it is with Chi Kung standing. When you stand to perform Chi Kung, it is not simply standing in the ordinary sense—you must stand very consciously aware.

When you begin the standing position, do not just stand—enter into this posture as if you are standing for the first time. Move into the position experiencing every element of your physical being. How do your feet, ankles, legs, and hips *feel?* As Chi Kung is an advanced level of human interaction with universal energy, truly knowing your body is the first step in entering into this mutual relationship.

The physical posture of Chi Kung standing involves your spine straight but not unnaturally forced into an erect position. Your legs are naturally separated at approximately shoulder level. Your knees are never locked, but allowed to bend very gently. Your arms are placed freely to your sides, your fingers loosely extended. Your gaze should be naturally forward, never unduly focused on any specific physical object.

Tongue, Teeth, and Eyes

When you perform Chi Kung exercises, your tongue should be lightly placed against the roof of your mouth. This causes the polarizing energies of your body, *Yin* and *Yang*, to meet and intermingle harmoniously. Your teeth should be allowed to lightly touch in a natural pattern.

Generally during Chi Kung your eyes will be gently closed. As you begin many of the exercises, however, keep your eyes open as you begin to take control and focus your mental energy. While doing this, it is important not to visually focus upon any specific physical object. As everything in this universe is composed of energy, you do not wish to take undue amounts of any undefined energy into your being prior to your Chi Kung practices. Thus, allow your eyes to randomly focus as your attention draws inward.

The Meridians

Chi permeates every aspect of every element of this universe. As such, Chi is present in every molecule of the human body. Though it is universally present in your being, it travels along exact pathways known in Chinese as *Jing*.

Jing, or as they are commonly referred to in English, "Meridians," are invisible channels inside your body that function in much the same way as your blood vessels. Whereas blood circulates throughout your entire body through your blood vessels, Chi travels via your Meridians.

Each organ of the human body has a Meridian that governs the flow of Chi to and from it. When you are in balance, your Meridian channels are open and Chi nourishes your organs and the various body functions they each individually affect. When you are out of balance your body shows symptoms of physical and emotional illness, which indicates one or more of your Meridians has become blocked.

The Constant Meridians

There are twelve "Constant Meridians" that function within each human body, referred to as such because Chi energy circulates through them in a constant and continually delineated path. Of these twelve, ten are defined by the specific organ of the human body that they dominate:

Dan Jing, "Gall Bladder Meridian"
Gan Jing, "Liver Meridian"
Fei Jing, "Lung Meridian"
Da Chang Jing, "Large Intestine Meridian"
Xian Chang Jing, "Small Intestine Meridian"
Wei Jing, "Stomach Meridian"
Pi Jing, "Spleen Meridian"
Xin Jing, "Heart Meridian"
Pang Guang Jing, "Bladder Meridian"
and *Shun Jing*, "Kidney Meridian"

The final two Constant Meridians, *Xin Bao Jing*, "Heart Constrictor Meridian," which regulates the sexual and reproductive Chi energy, and *Sao Jian Jing*, "Triple Warmer Meridian," which dominates three specific functions of the body: the energy of respiration, the control of digestion, and the control of bodily discharges, are related to the control of bodily functions.

Each of these Constant Meridians possesses a location on both the right and left sides of your body. By practicing Chi Kung, your Meridians are stimulated and thus remain balanced and open with a constant flow of Chi travelling through them (see Figure 1.1, following page).

The Secondary Meridians

There are two additional Meridians that also aid in the control and circulation of Chi throughout your body. These Secondary Meridians influence highly specific Chi channels and bodily activities. Thus they are referred to as "Secondary Meridians." They are the "Conceptual Meridian," which is responsible for balancing the overall functioning of your body, and the "Governing Vessel Meridian," which nourishes and aligns the other Meridians.

Chi and Your Environment

The benefits you will gain from Chi Kung are directly related to the physical environment where you practice, the type of food you eat, and your lifestyle. If you are in a noisy, dirty, or polluted environment, eating bad food, drinking

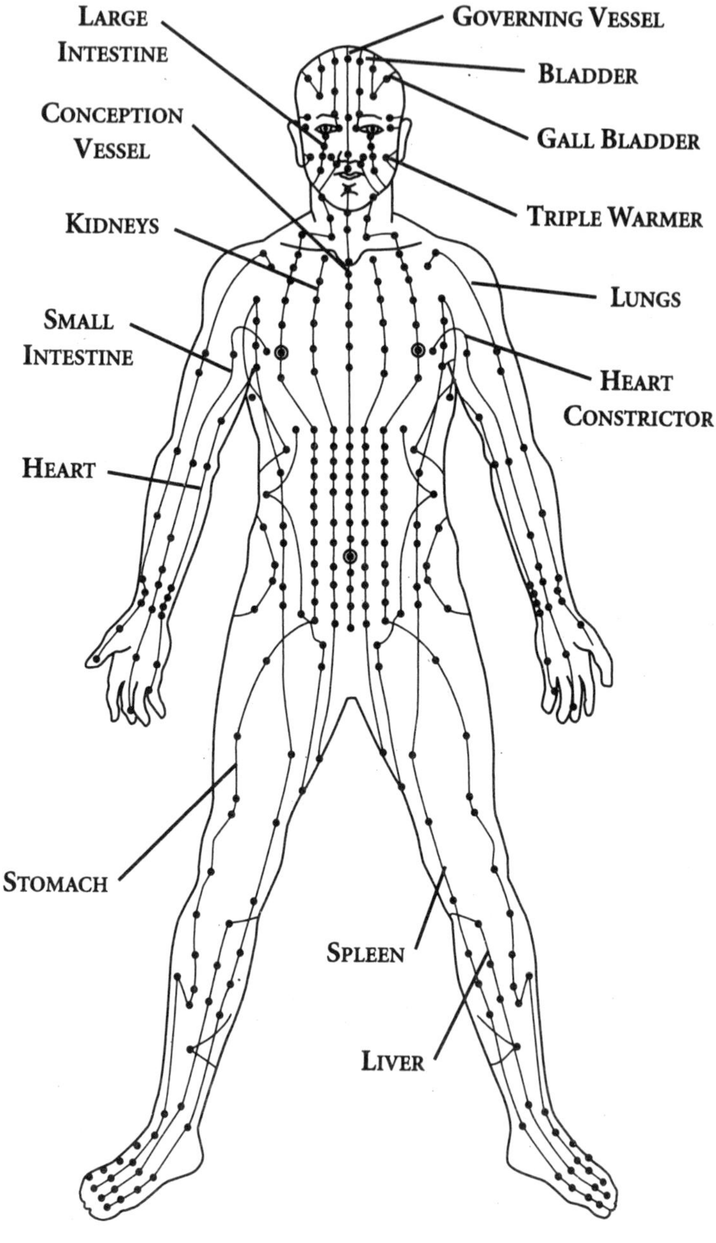

1.1 The Energy Meridians

bad drink (such as alcohol or soft drinks), and associating with negative people, your mind will not only be unduly distracted, but your physical body will be suffering due to your impure surroundings.

As you begin on your path to Chi consciousness, it is essential to know that you are in control of your life. Therefore, you can focus your energy and move your body to any place you desire. Allow the Chi Kung techniques in this book to help you focus your life and move you to a placement and position where all the positive energy of the universe can embellish you.

Chi and Personal Power

Chi Kung is a process of body-and-mind purification and enhancement, not a method to direct excess amounts of Chi into your body so that you can physically or mentally overpower others. Do not practice it with the hopes of gaining some mythical power to dominate others, or your practice will be fruitless.

There is a natural balance in this universe. If any person attempts to gain or maintain control over another, this balance is set out of alignment and the power-seeking individual quickly falls from their superior position. For this reason, the pure Chi Kung practitioner only practices the exercises as a means of coming into a more conscious interaction with the universe's positive energies. From this they can help all of humanity move to a more conscious plane of divine interaction.

chapter two

Tiao Chi

Tiao Chi is translated from the Chinese as "The Harmonizing of the Breath." Breath is what brings Chi into your body. When you refine your breathing techniques to an exacting science, enhanced amounts of Chi can be consciously taken into your being to aid you in times of physical or mental need.

The Tiao Chi exercise is the first preliminary breathing technique you must learn before attempting to perform any other forms of Chi Kung. In this exercise, your breath and your body are brought into conscious harmony and universal Chi may enter and travel through your being unhindered.

Chi Blockage

It is necessary to perform this exercise before proceeding further with Chi Kung because if there is any hindrance to the flow of Chi along any Meridian channel in your body, the enhanced intake of Chi may reach an impasse point causing a Chi buildup in that specific bodily region. This can have an injurious effect to the overall Chi flow throughout your entire being.

The factors that have the potential to develop a Chi blockage are: the long-term intake of improper food or drink, breathing polluted air over an extended time, an unhealed injury to a specific bodily part, or an underexercised, aging body. If Chi blockage has occurred, it means that you are out of balance with nature. Thus, if you perform Chi Kung before removing this blockage, the potential is substantially heightened that you will be thrown further out of balance with the specific Yin or Yang energy common to your obstructed Meridian and freeing that blockage will become more complicated.

For this reason, Tiao Chi is always performed prior to more advanced Chi Kung practices in order to open your Meridian pathways and allow Chi to enter and successfully flow throughout your being, unhindered. Due to the very subtle and effective nature of this technique it is often times referred to as *Tong Guan,* or "Opening the Gate."

Tiao Chi Exercise One

To begin the Tiao Chi exercise, stand up and loosen your body by moving your arms and legs around slowly and naturally—twist your ankles and wrists from side to side and pivot your neck. This will relieve any minor pent-up muscle tension you may have and cause blood circulation to increase throughout your entire body.

Once this is accomplished, sit on the floor in Lotus Posture. As discussed, if the cross-legged posture is uncomfortable, you can perform this exercise by sitting in a chair with your spine erect.

Once you have settled into your seated posture, close your eyes and become comfortable with your body—simply mentally relax into your position.

Sitting Consciously

Many people sit down with the intention of immediately entering into a meditative Chi Kung technique and attempt to mentally force themselves immediately into the exercise. What this does is cause your adrenal gland to release hormones that cause your heart rate to increase and your mind to become alert and active—the exact opposite of what you wish to achieve in this exercise. Therefore, never force yourself to sit down and expect to immediately enter into a meditative mindset. Instead, take a few moments to become comfortable with your position.

Once you feel that you are mentally ready, consciously breathe in deeply through your nose—feel your lungs and stomach expand with the inhalation. This inhalation should not be unnaturally forced, but should, nonetheless, cause your lungs to fill completely, thereby expanding your chest and stomach. Once your in-breath is completed, the Chi-filled oxygen should be allowed to leave your lungs naturally, exiting through your mouth. Perform this deep-breathing exercise by taking air in through your nose and allowing it to be exhaled through your mouth for seven complete breath cycles.

Deep Breathing

Deep breathing is one of the most basic and fundamental things you can do to not only instantly revitalize yourself with Chi, but to cleanse your lungs from the pollutants of the modern world. Additionally, the initial deep inhalation of new fresh air in the Tiao Chi exercise performs the task of cleansing the body's Meridian pathways. This is because the human body is in a constant pattern of taking in vital Chi through the breath in the same rhythmic pattern hour-after-hour, day-after-day. Throughout your life, you breathe in a constant pattern; thus, your body becomes accustomed to a specific level of Chi entering your being with each breath cycle. By inhaling deeply, you instantly change this pattern and your body becomes alive with excessive amounts of Chi. Your Meridian pathways are instantaneously purged from any blockage that may have resulted from the stagnation of Chi.

Tiao Chi Exercise Two

Upon the completion of the initial stage of Tiao Chi, you will want to immediately continue forward with the second stage of this exercise, where you focus your meditative attention upon your breath. This is quite simple. Breathe calmly in through your nose. As the breath enters your body, be aware of its life-giving force, travelling naturally through your nose, down into your lungs. When it is time to exhale, do so naturally through your mouth.

At this stage of Chi Kung, no element of your breath is forced or controlled. You simply observe the Chi-filled energy of life naturally entering and exiting your body. The breath comes in, it goes out—you come to realize that you are only an earthly conduit for this divine process of Chi transmission. A new breath comes in, you witness it. It goes out, you witness it. Allow yourself to simply be.

Perform this phase of the exercise for as long as you feel necessary. As it is a very focusing and meditative process, so it should go on for at least seven natural breath cycles, but can go on for much longer. Once you have completed this stage of Tiao Chi you can move forward with additional Chi Kung exercises, or simply encounter the day in a much more profoundly aware state.

chapter three

Dan Tien

Dan Tien is a term coined by ancient Taoist monks to describe the most important location on the human body in relation to conscious interaction with Chi. In Chinese, *Dan Tien* means "Field of Elixir."

This understanding has been adopted and used by many facets of Asian culture. To the acupuncturist, this location is designated by the expression *Quhai,* translated as "Sea of Chi." In the Korean language it is *Tan Jun,* and in Japanese the word *Hara* is used to define this same bodily location.

Hara is perhaps the word that is most commonly known when describing this location on the human body. This is due to that fact of its frequent usage in association with Aikido, and the Japanese martial arts in general.

Understanding the Dan Tien

Dan Tien is located on the human body where Chi congregates and can be accessed and used by the individual. Thus, this location is highly revered.

It is an absolute necessity that you become acutely aware of its location so you may become consciously interactive with Chi. Thus, your first step in active Chi Kung is to become interactive with your Dan Tien.

Defining Dan Tien

Dan Tien is located approximately two inches below your navel. From a central point it goes out approximately two inches in each direction. In addition to being the location where Chi congregates in your body, it is your body's center of gravity. For this reason, martial artists become highly aware of this energy center through practicing their advanced form of movement. In fact, whenever you hear a martial artist let out a yell as they unleash a technique it signifies they are releasing Chi energy along with their movement.

Martial artists are not the only individuals who can become sharply aware of their Dan Tien. This knowledge is available to anyone who places the proper focus upon this energy center. To achieve this interactive knowledge, you must initially perform a few simple movements that will help you define it. From this, you can move forward with

Chi Kung and consciously bring Chi into all the movements of your everyday life.

Dan Tien Defining Exercise One

Begin by standing in a natural position with your arms loosely at your side. Keep your spine erect, but not stiff. Move your neck around a little bit, releasing any tension. Do the same with your shoulders.

When you feel comfortable, close your eyes. Slowly become very conscious of your body. This process should not be forced. Do not attempt to strain your mind, telling yourself, "Be conscious—be conscious." As you progress through several sessions with this exercise and other Chi Kung techniques presented in this book, you will come to a state of refined interactive consciousness with your body. You will find that it is a very natural process to become intuitively focused upon specific components of your being. Therefore, at the early states of your Chi Kung, never force your body or mind—simply begin to develop your new interrelationship with your body.

Body Consciousness

If this is your first endeavor into body consciousness, simply begin to take notice of how your body feels. First place your concentration on your feet. Ask yourself, "How do they feel?" Then your legs. Move up to your torso, consciously taking notice of each inch of your body. Experience your arms, and finally your neck and head.

At the point you have taken inventory of all these bodily locations, begin to focus your concentration on the approximate location of your Dan Tien. Begin by mentally surveying this area of your body, which you have probably placed very little focus upon previously.

As the exact location of Dan Tien is unique to each individual, it is *you* who must locate Dan Tien in your own body. Thus, simply begin to mentally feel this region.

As your consciousness becomes more focused on this energy center, begin to witness your breathing through your nose. Feel it enter your body, providing you with life-sustaining oxygen. Then witness it exiting your body through your mouth. Do this for a few natural breath cycles and then begin to mentally send your breaths to your Dan Tien—visualize each in-breath traveling through your nose, deep into your body, and lighting up your Dan Tien with golden Chi-filled energy.

Do not elongate these breaths for an unnatural period of time. Simply allow them to travel in and out of your body naturally. Each breath enters, touches your Dan Tien with golden Chi-filled energy and then exits through your mouth.

After you have performed this segment of the exercise for approximately seven natural breath cycles—with your next in breath, again, watch it travel to your Dan Tien. Once this in-breath has been completed, hold it locked into your Dan Tien for approximately seven seconds. Then, release it naturally through your mouth. Do this segment of the exercise for approximately seven natural breath cycles and then return to normal breathing for a few minutes before you open your eyes and finish this exercise.

With the practice of this simple technique, you are consciously causing Chi energy to activate in your Dan Tien. You will begin to develop an understanding of this vital energy center.

Dan Tien Defining Exercise Two

Stand in a natural stance as you did with Dan Tien Defining Exercise One. Loosen up your body and settle into a focused mental state with your eyes closed. Breathe naturally; consciously experience golden Chi-filled breaths entering and invigorating your body.

When you feel you are mentally ready, focus your attention on your Dan Tien and be aware of your breaths traveling to and from this energy center through your nose. After approximately seven natural breath cycles, bend your elbows, and bring your hands up to waist level at the frontal region of your body. As you do this, allow the inner tips of your fingers to come into light contact with your thumb.

In acupuncture it is understood that several Meridians culminate in the tips of your fingers. By joining your fingers and thumb together in this fashion, you seal off any Chi that may be randomly exiting your body, thus maintaining a more constant circulation of Chi.

As you take your next breath, be aware of it entering your body through your nose and traveling to your Dan Tien in a golden light. As it flows inward, allow your knees to lightly bend. As you bend, simultaneously pull your hands back at waist level until they reach your mid-region as you complete your in-breath.

Hold this Chi breath in your body for approximately seven seconds, visualizing the golden light of Chi energy emanating from your Dan Tien and expanding forward in front of your body.

When you are ready to exhale, do so slowly. As your breath exits you body via your mouth, see it illuminating the area around your body in the form of golden Chi-filled light. As you exhale, simultaneously bring your knees and your hands slowly back to their original position. When your breath has been completely exhaled, do not breathe in for approximately seven seconds. Instead, experience the lightness of Chi-filled energy throughout your body.

After this interval, again breathe in your Chi-filled breath, as your body slowly lowers and your hands pull back, exposing your Dan Tien, which is emanating Chi from this powerful energy center (see Figures 3.1–3.4, following page).

This exercise should be performed for a maximum of seven cycles per training session. You will not only come to effectively define the exact location of your Dan Tien, but you will additionally experience how Chi can be brought into your body and then projected into the environment around you.

The Three Dan Tiens

To the modern practitioner of Chi Kung, there is a single focal point that is the primary focus of Chi interaction, the Dan Tien. In ancient times, however, there were in fact, three Dan Tiens that were accessed by the Chi Kung practitioner.

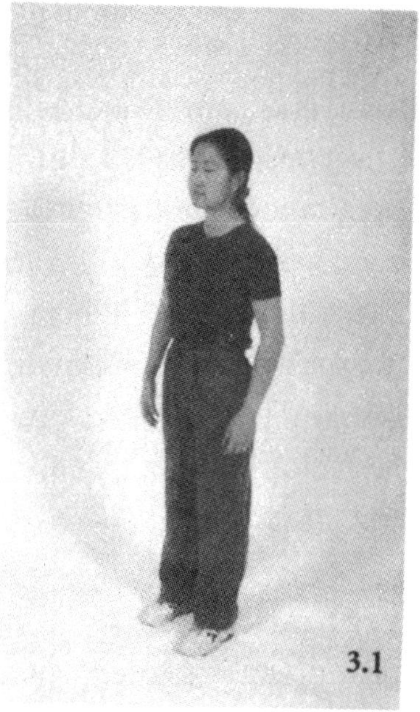

3.1

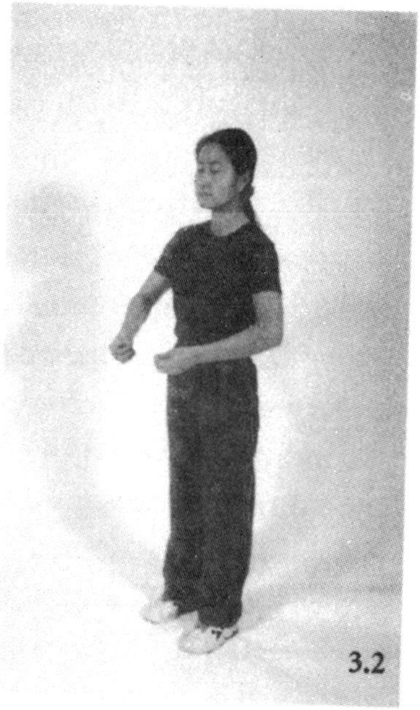

3.2

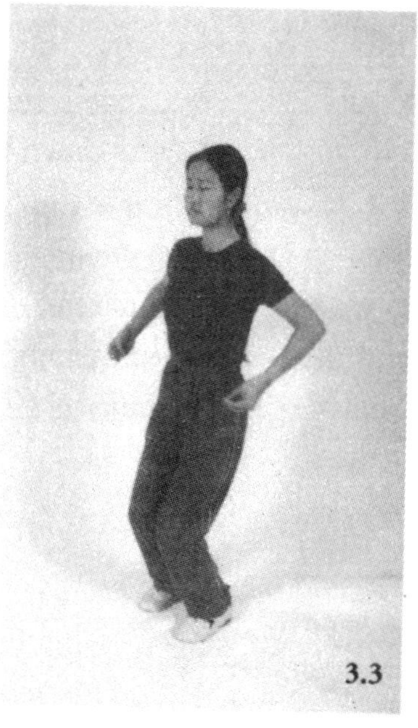

3.3

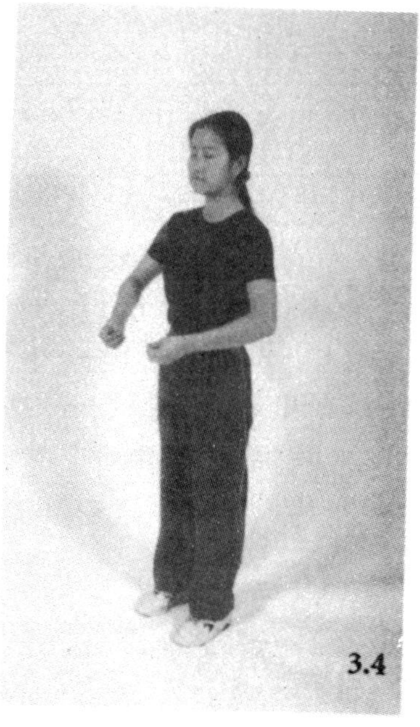

3.4

This understanding was known as *San Dan Tien,* or the "Three Fields of Cultivation."

The first of these three Dan Tiens is the one detailed previously. Since ancient times, it has been known that this Dan Tien was the place in the body where Chi energy congregated, and could be drawn upon when needed.

The second, or middle, Dan Tien (known in Chinese as *Zhong Dan Tien*) is located at the solar plexus. This energy center was believed to be responsible for proper breathing. An individual who focused his Chi-oriented meditation upon this Dan Tien was believed to possess superior strength and unequaled endurance.

The third of these three energy centers is the *Zuigao,* or the "Upper Dan Tien." This focal point is located at the pineal gland, commonly called the "Third Eye." Chi meditation upon this Dan Tien was known to provide the individual with superior mental skills.

Though the primary focal point for the Chi Kung practitioner is the Dan Tien located just below the navel, the two additional Dan Tiens are important energy centers that can be cultivated to access specific types of Chi. Therefore, these bodily locations must be embraced for the student of Chi Kung to come to an overall mastery of this science. In the following pages, we will detail Chi Kung techniques that activate all three of the Dan Tiens.

chapter four

Tao Yin

Tao Yin, literally translated from the Chinese, means "Stretching and Contracting the Body." In practice, Tao Yin is the technique for seven ancient exercises that dissipate Chi obstructions from your body.

Since ancient times, Tao Yin has been understood to not only invigorate the body with Chi, but to prolong life and promise immortality. This is due to the fact that the seven exercises relieve the body of illnesses, while invigorating it with Chi.

Tao Yin is additionally understood to focus the mind to the degree where the practitioner can master advanced techniques of Chi breath control and meditation.

Tao Yin is made up of highly exacting Chi purification techniques. The seven exercises that make up Tao Yin must be performed in a continual sequence, in order that all Meridians of your body are stimulated and cleared of any potential blockage.

When the seven Tao Yin exercises are performed, the inhalation and exhalation of breath must be done in an acutely focused manner. While practicing these exercises you cannot allow the physical aspects of your body's movement to overpower your mental intent or the process of Chi infusion will not be actualized.

Tao Yin Exercise One: Kou Ch'ih

Translated from the Chinese, *Kou Ch'ih* means "Chattering of the Teeth." Kou Ch'ih is not only the primary Tao Yin exercise, but it is the preliminary exercise that, in ancient times, was performed before all other Chi Kung techniques due to its ability to nurture the brain and the body with necessary internal nutrients.

To correctly perform Kou Ch'ih, begin by closing your eyes and consciously encountering the vast abyss that exists in your own mental darkness. Mindfully embrace the understanding that within your own being is the link to divine consciousness, and the darkness that you see should not be feared—it is a pathway to self discovery, where you cannot only discover your meditative mind, but Ming ("Enlightenment") too.

With your eyes closed, take a few moments to engage the darkness. When you feel it is time, place your mental focus on your breath and begin to breathe slowly and naturally for seven cycles—inhaling and exhaling through your nose. Feel the life-giving breath entering and exiting your body.

Do not force your breath or mentally send it to any location within your body; simply observe the cosmic perfection of this process as your diaphragm expands with each in-breath, filling your lungs with life-giving oxygen and Chi, and contracting with each out-breath, leaving you with a sense of fulfilled lightness.

Upon the exhalation of the seventh breath, consciously direct all of the remaining air out of your lungs, allowing them to become completely empty. Accomplish this by contracting your upper abdomen muscles. Witness the feeling you experience as the final Chi-filled breath exits your body through your mouth, leaving your being embraced in Chi-saturated lightness.

Do not immediately breathe in again, but begin to lightly bring your teeth together. Do not grind them; simply gently expand your jaw, with your lips remaining closed, and bring your upper teeth down upon your bottom teeth thirty-six times. At first, the lack of air in your lungs may cause you emotional discomfort. If you must breathe during the thirty-six teeth chatterings, do so calmly and naturally through your nose.

No Chi-refining technique should cause you physical or emotional discomfort. This is especially the case with Tao Yin. Therefore, do not force any exercise; if you need to breathe, move, or reposition yourself to regain you physical or mental comfort, do so without hesitation.

As you move forward with Chi Kung techniques, it will become more and more natural for your lungs to remain without oxygen for extended periods of time. This is due to the fact that as you become increasingly filled with expanded amounts of Chi, you will learn to gain mastery over the repetitive elements of your physical being and they will no longer dominate your existence.

While practicing Kou Ch'ih, you should also not attempt to rush through the thirty-six movements of teeth chattering in order to breathe again, as this disrupts the meditative focusing involved in this Chi exercise. Simply allow your teeth to meet each other thirty-six times in a constant and steady pattern.

When you have completed the thirty-sixth teeth chattering, breathe in slowly and naturally through your nose. Experience the power of this Chi-filled breath embracing your being.

Seated Kou Ch'ih

Kou Ch'ih is ideally practiced in a seated posture when it is used as a primary Chi-focusing technique prior to additional seated Chi Kung techniques. However, when it is used along with the other six Tao Yin exercises it is more appropriately performed standing. This is because six of the seven Tao Yin exercises are dependent upon a standing posture, making it much more conducive to the constant flow of Chi to not sit and then rise between these practices.

Standing Kou Ch'ih

To perform Kou Ch'ih from a standing posture, simply stand with your feet naturally separated at shoulder-level. Your arms should lay loosely at your side. Then simply perform the teeth-chattering exercise as previously described.

Kou Ch'ih and Yu Chiang

The ancient practice of Kou Ch'ih was designed to stimulate the body's production of *Yu Chiang,* or "saliva." To the Taoists, saliva is known as "Liquid Jade." From a physiological standpoint, saliva is believed to be one of the most nourishing elements produced within the human body. It is believed to feed the brain and moisten the *Wu Tsang,* "The Five Organs": lungs, heart, pancreas, kidneys, and liver. It is understood that spitting is one of the worst things an individual can do because it unnecessarily wastes this vital liquid.

Tun To

Tun To is the ancient Taoist Chi practice of slowly and consciously swallowing the saliva, thereby fostering the continued health of the body and allowing Chi to move freely within it. Upon the completion of Kou Ch'ih, the saliva that has been produced should be circulated around the mouth. Once this has been accomplished, Tun To has been performed.

Ancient Traditions—Modern Science

To the modern individual, the thought that saliva is a nurturing element to the whole body is often times immediately dismissed as ancient superstition. However, when one experiences the practice of Chi Kung, one rapidly understands that though some of the techniques may be rooted in timeworn traditions, the physical and mental exhilaration instantly provides the insight that though modern science may provide clearer physiological definitions of biological actions, the ancient Chi-development exercises still prove that energy is, in fact, developed and cultivated when the techniques are practiced.

It is imperative, then, to never simply dismiss any ancient Taoist Chi Kung technique simply because it may seem somewhat absurd when based in modern scientific analysis. Though these practices may be thousands of years old, they would not have continued to be used had they not provided results. With personal exploration and performance, you will experience that each step of each practice/exercise fills you with the empowerment of Chi.

Tao Yin Exercise Two

The second Tao Yin exercise is known as "The Ocean Churns As You Swallow Its Essence." To perform this technique, stand in a loose and natural posture. Close your eyes and take in a few natural breaths, inhaling through your nose and exhaling through your mouth. Be aware of these breaths traveling to and emanating from your Dan Tien.

After a few moments of Dan Tien breath meditation, begin to very consciously feel your body, starting at your feet. Is there any tension? If there is, move them slightly as you watch golden Chi traveling from your Dan Tien down your leg to embrace and revitalize them. Then, place your feet firmly back upon the ground. Direct your consciousness to your ankles. If there is any discomfort, move them around slowly as you direct Chi to them. Move your consciousness up your legs, truly experiencing them. If you experience any lack of comfort, breathe Chi into them. Feel your hands. Any pressure? Move them slightly and send them Chi. Allow your consciousness to travel up your torso, feeling your neck and head. If any bodily location is experiencing an uneasy feeling, move it slightly, causing added blood circulation, and then very consciously breathe Chi from your Dan Tien to that location.

Remember, Chi is endless. All you need to do is breathe in its power and you will be re-energized. Once you have become very consciously in tune with your body, "The Ocean Churns As You Swallow Its Essence" continues by taking in a deep breath through your nose and watching it travel to your Dan Tien in a golden flow. Once the breath has completely entered your Dan Tien, you hold it in place and begin to circulate your tongue around your closed mouth ten times. At the completion of the tenth cycle, place your tongue firmly against your palate and release the gold breath of Chi through your nose. Witness it encompassing your body.

You will have noticed that excess saliva is being produced in your mouth. When it is time to breathe again, do so naturally, bringing the breath in through your nose. As the in-breath is completed, allow this excess saliva to be slowly swallowed nourishing your entire being. It will take approximately three natural breath cycles to consciously perform this Tun To exercise.

By performing this third element of the Tao Yin, you will have accomplished *Tai Shih,* or "Feeding of the Embryo." This expression details that your inner being is flushed with Chi.

Tao Yin Exercise Three

The third stage of Tao Yin is known as "Turning the Heavenly Pillar." To begin this exercise, keep your eyes closed and consciously take in one deep breath through your nose. Witness this breath traveling to your Dan Tien and filling it with golden Chi energy. Lock this breath in this positioning for a moment, embracing its power. When you feel that it is necessary, naturally release this Chi breath through your mouth. With your next in-breath, taken in through your nose, guide the breath toward your Dan Tien, open your eyes, bring your palms together in front of you body, with your left hand facing upward, your right hand facing downward—allow them to meet just in front of your solar plexus. Keep your feet in a stationary position, pointing naturally forward, and turn your upper torso toward the right from waist level. As you reach your maximum pivot, while keeping your spine erect, guide your shoulders a little farther to the right than is natural for you. Consciously embrace this upper-body stretch.

As you perform this movement, allow your eyes to look as far to your left as possible without actually moving your head. When it comes time to release your in-breath, do so, bringing your body and eyes back to their natural, central position.

With your next natural in-breath, turn your body in the same fashion to the left, allowing your eyes to look to the extreme right. Release the breath when it is time and return to your central position. This movement should be performed seven times in association with each new in-breath.

The purpose of this exercise, from a physical standpoint, is to stimulate your Meridian pathways through a technique of movement that is natural, yet slightly exaggerated. From a more metaphysical perspective, this exercise moves the body in one direction, while the eyes and their vision travel in the opposite. What this serves to symbolize is that within all Yang there is the element of Yin—as within all Yin there is Yang. Your two hands remain touching one another to center and intermingle the Yin and the Yang, thus grounding your being in the balance of the two primary energies of this universe (see Figures 4.1–4.6, pages 36–37).

Tao Yin Exercise Four

Tao Yin Exercise Four begins by rubbing your hands together to make them warm. Do not simply do this without awareness of what is actually taking place. As all Chi development exercises are based in mental science, you must make all Chi Kung a very conscious process of your mental evolution. To this end, close your eyes and breathe in naturally through

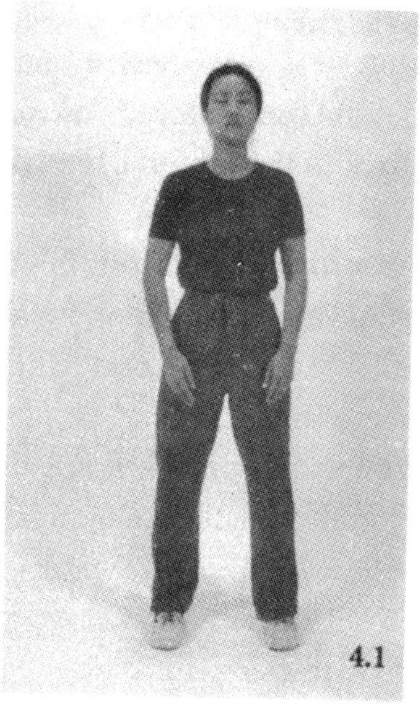
4.1

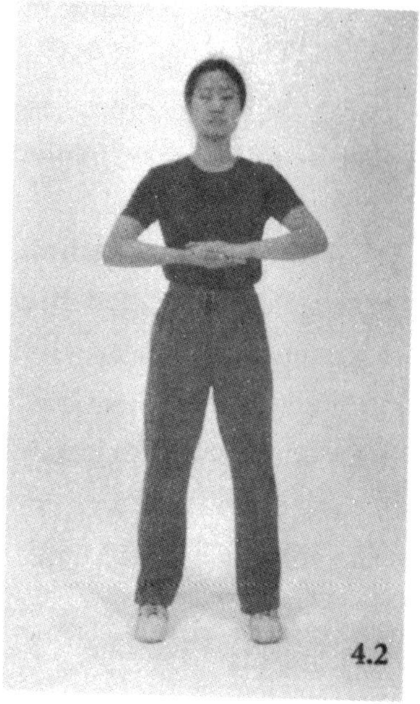
4.2

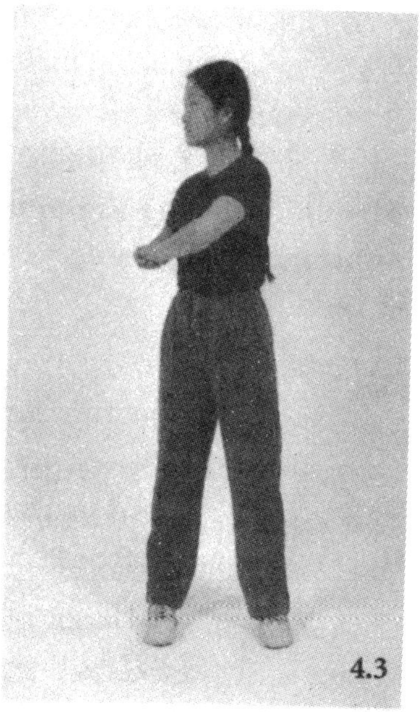
4.3

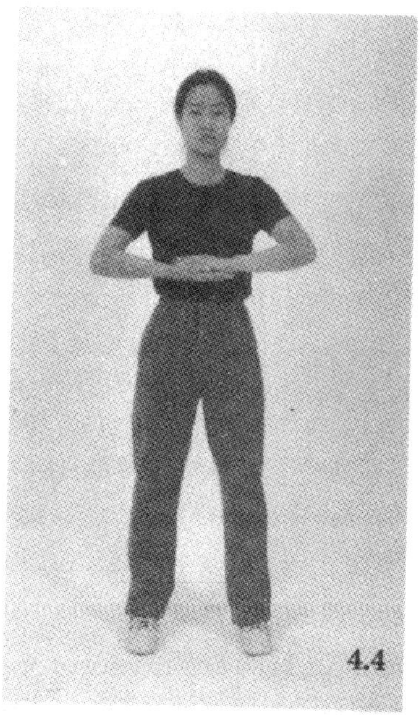
4.4

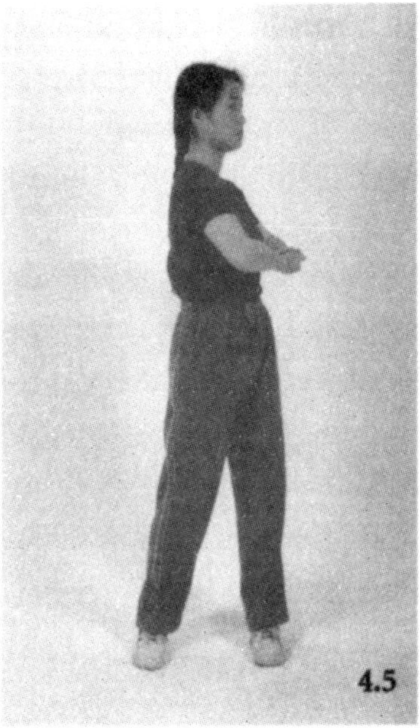

4.5

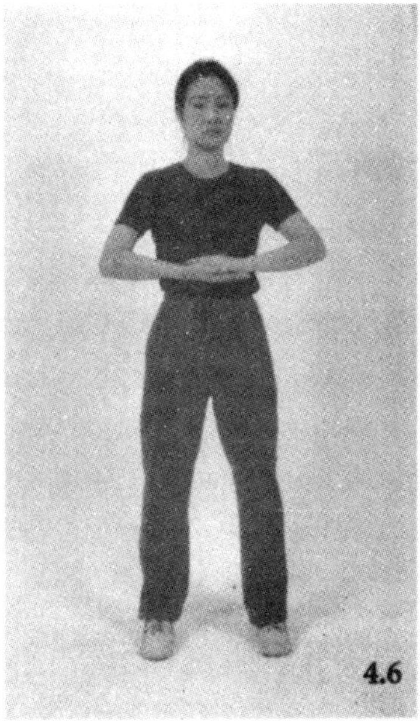

4.6

your nose as you gently rub your hands together. With each new in-breath, visualize the golden light of Chi traveling in through your nose and progressing to your hands, as they become illuminated with the golden essence of Chi.

At the point your hands have become warm and invigorated with Chi, generally after three-to-five breath cycles, place your left hand on your Dan Tien and your right hand on your forehead. For a moment, embrace the Chi-filled warmth your hands reveal upon these bodily locations. With your next in-breath, begin to lightly rub the area around your Dan Tien with your left hand. Experience how your hand, rubbing this region, dissipates any Chi that may be stagnating, and witness it expanding throughout your entire body.

After you have completed one single in-breath and out-breath, stop rubbing. Take one more natural in-breath through your nose, feel it expand your lungs with Chi-filled air. Allow this breath to naturally leave your body through your nose.

With your next in-breath, begin to rub your forehead. Experience how the Chi energy locked in your Third Eye (Zuigao) is released throughout your body. At the completion of one natural in-breath and one natural out-breath, allow both of your hands to return to natural positions on your side. Take a few moments for natural breathing, experiencing the Chi radiating throughout your body (see Figures 4.7–4.10, following page).

Tao Yin Exercise Five

Keeping your eyes closed, bring your consciousness to your breath and progress through three natural breath cycles—witness golden Chi traveling to your Dan Tien and radiating throughout your body from this location. When you have completed the third exaltation, bring your hands together and again, along with your Chi-conscious breath, rub them together in front of you until they are suitably warmed up. When you have completed this process, bring your hands around your back and place them upon your kidney region.

As your kidneys are elementally important organs to the proper functioning of your body, and are understood to be very important in the proper circulation of Chi, they, too, must be freed from any potential obstructions so that Chi

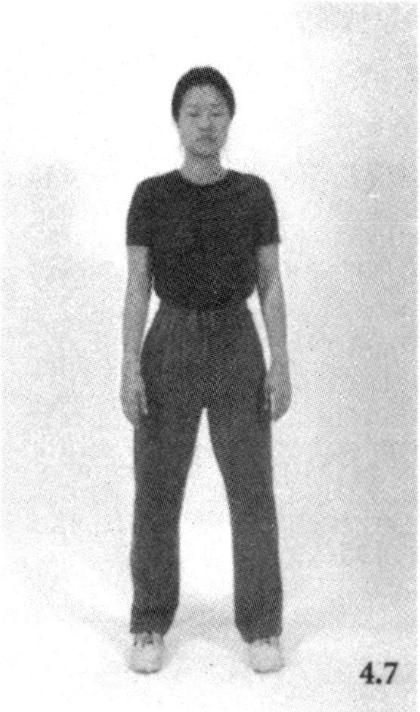

4.7

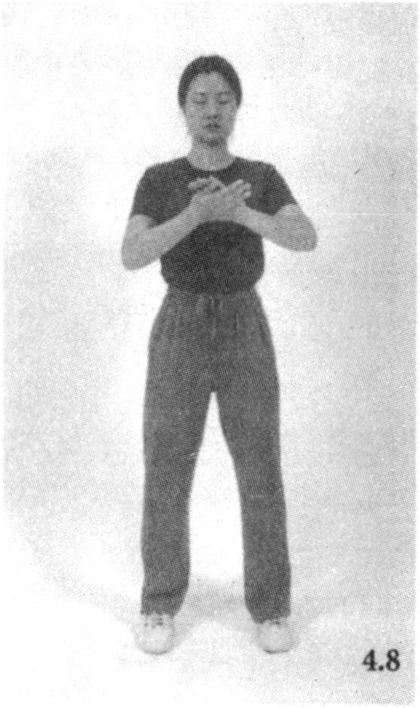

4.8

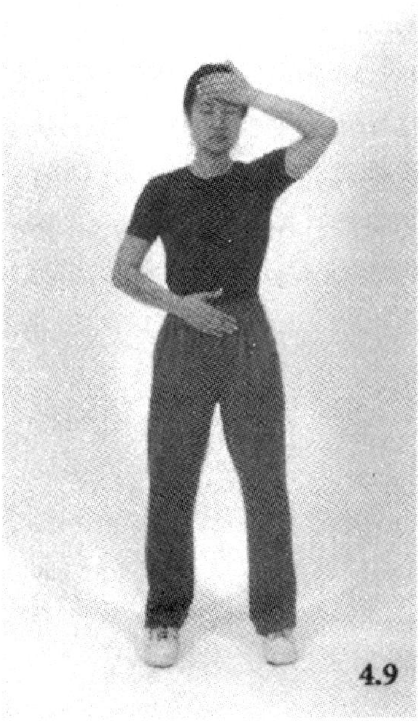

4.9

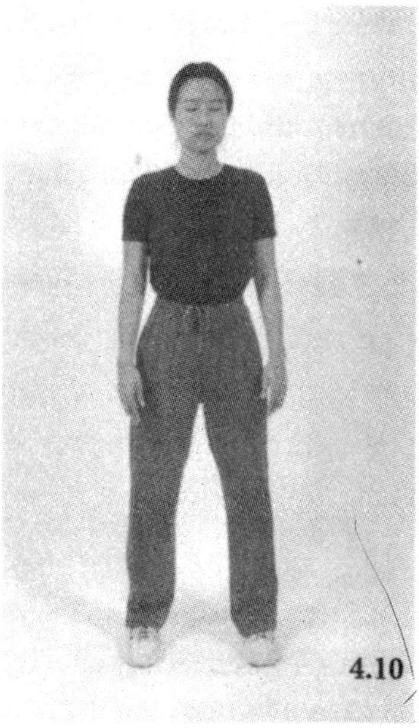

4.10

can flow unhindered throughout your being. With your warm hands, rub them in an up-and-down motion thirty-six times in the kidney region of your back. Breathe naturally as you witness, with each in-breath, golden Chi flowing in through your nose, traveling down your arms and embracing your kidneys with the freeing energy of golden Chi light. Exhale each out-breath through your mouth.

When you have completed this procedure, bring your hands back to your side, breathe naturally, and embrace the continually evolving freedom your ethereal body is encountering (see Figures 4.11–4.14, following page).

Tao Yin Exercise Six

After a few moments of meditative reflection after finishing Tao Yin Exercise Five, again bring your consciousness to your breath, breathe in Chi though your nose, and send it down your arms as you rub your hands together for a third time. Once they are suitably filled with Chi, place your warm hands on the back of your head, with your palms covering your ears. Allow your fingers to extend around the back of your skull. Focus your consciousness on your breath as you breathe in a natural and deep Chi-filled breath through your nose. When the in-breath is complete, lock it in your Dan Tien. At the same time, begin to lightly tap your forefingers on the rear of your skull, close to your spine. This tapping should be performed for a total of thirty-six repetitions, thus, relieving any Chi blockage that may have occurred along your spine and in your cranium.

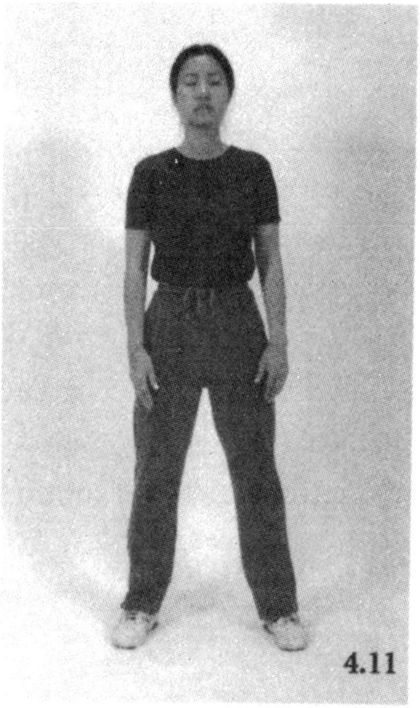

4.11

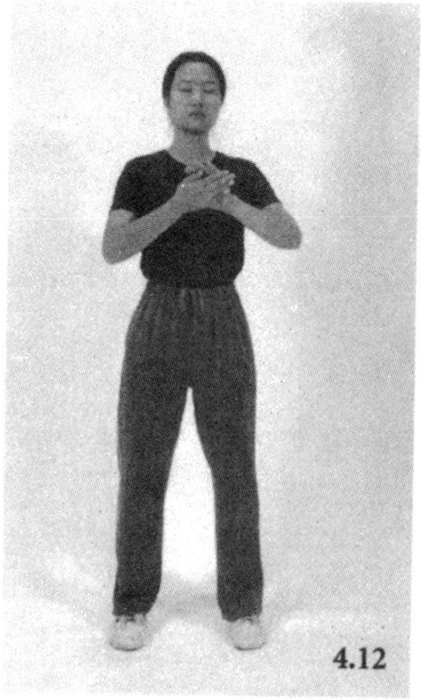

4.12

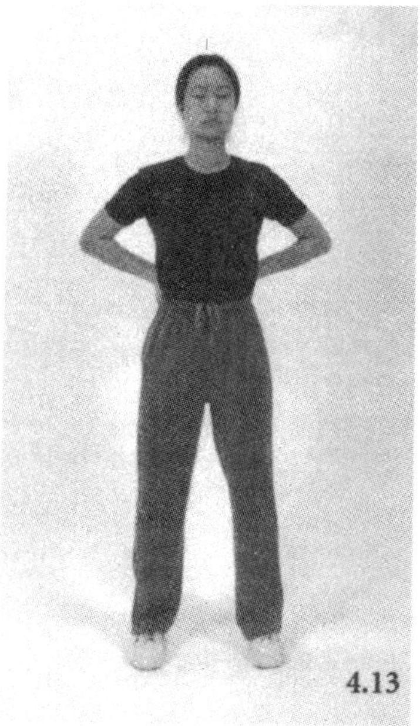

4.13

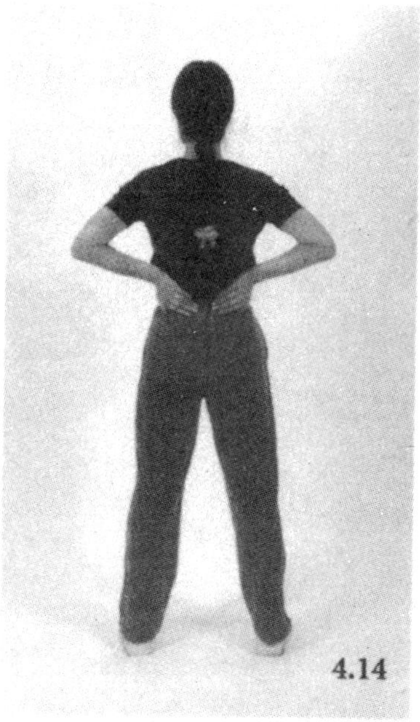

4.14

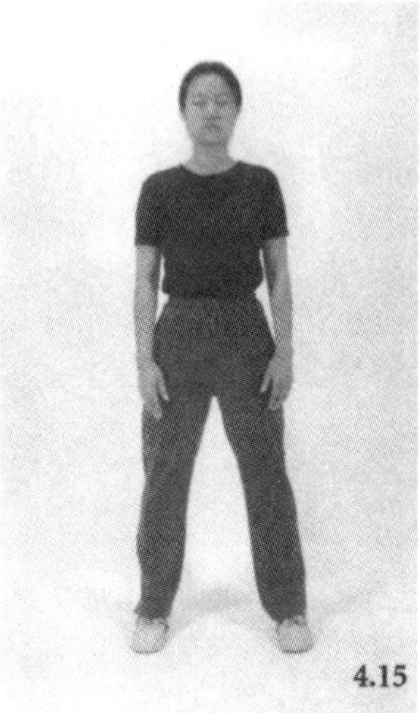

4.15

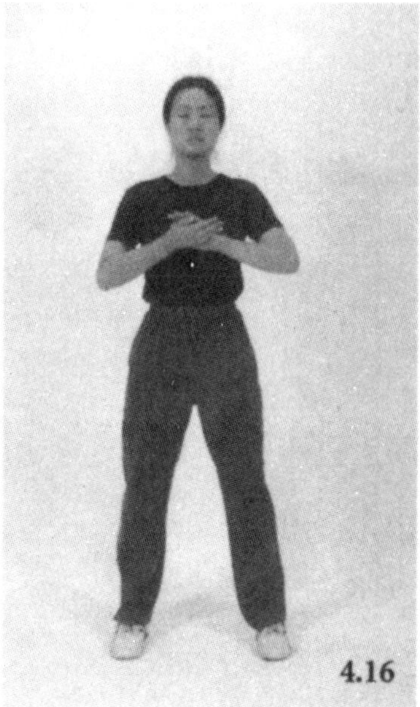

4.16

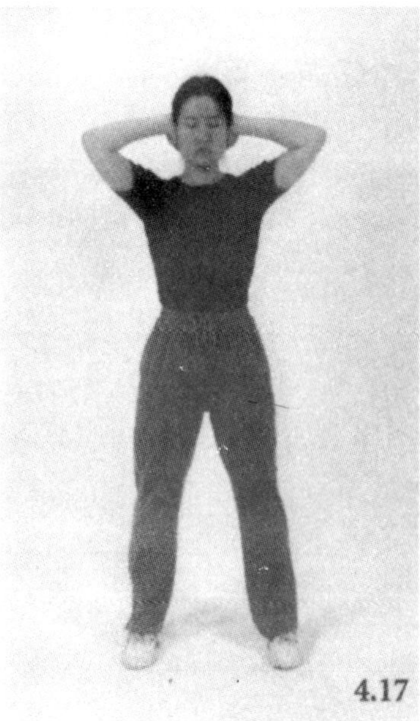

4.17

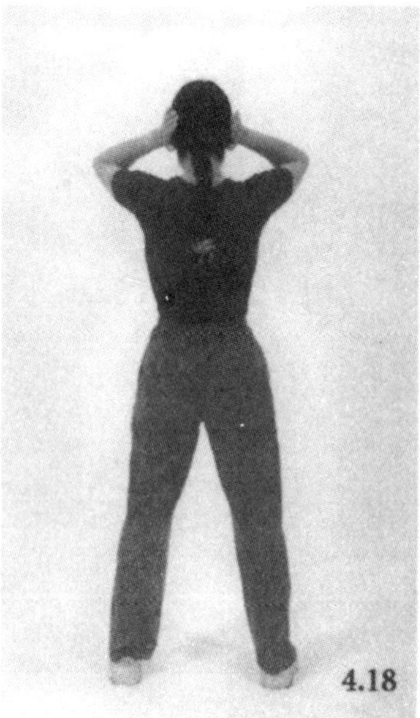

4.18

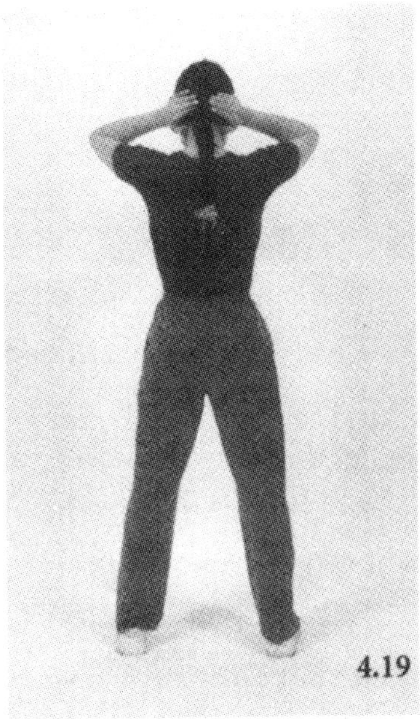

4.19

Upon the completion of the thirty-sixth tap, return your hands to your side and meditatively breathe naturally (see Figures 4.15–4.19, page 42, and above).

Your Hands and Tao Yin

The Chi-filled rubbing of your hands in Tao Yin is performed so that you very consciously send Chi to your hands. This helps in the removal of Meridian blockages that may have occurred in your body. The same techniques of Tao Yin that you perform on your own body can additionally be used when you perform acupressure, or massage another individual to help remove Chi blockage in his or her body. Therefore, the techniques of Tao Yin are not only beneficial to enhanced Chi flow throughout your body, but can additionally benefit others, too.

Tao Yin Exercise Seven

Your eyes remain closed as you progress into the seventh stage of Tao Yin, known as "Bringing in the Double Wind." As your common Chi-blockage locations have been freed by this point in your Tao Yin experience, it has therefore become much easier for you to successfully bring excess amounts of Chi into your body and have it flow unhindered. Thus, it is now time to not only clear any final blockage points, but to invigorate your entire physical being and surroundings with positive Chi energy.

Begin by breathing a few natural breath cycles. When you feel you are ready, consciously exhale. As you do so, extend your arms to their full length, parallel to the ground, in front of your body. Your hands should be open and your palms facing one another at approximately a one-foot separation. When it is time for you to inhale, do so powerfully, with focused determination. As this Chi breath enters your body, through your nose, see it dynamically traveling to your Dan Tien. As you breathe in, simultaneously make your hands into fists and draw them toward you as if you were pulling a heavy object into your body.

After completing the in-breath, feel the power of Chi emanating from your Dan Tien, and physically enhancing your physical being and the external space around you.

Embrace this Chi power as you slowly, mentally count to ten. Upon ten, release this breath through your mouth, as your fists release and your arms travel outward toward their original extended position. Once they have reached this level, allow your lungs to remain consciously empty for the same count of ten. Experience how your body surges with Chi energy and your surroundings are vibrating with the Chi energy emanating from your body.

At the count of ten, again breathe in Chi-filled air as you perform this technique for a second time—making your hands into fists as they pull that large object toward your body and your entire being becomes filled with Chi. Once this action has been completed, again count to ten, releasing the breath in the same pattern.

Tao Yin Seven should be performed a maximum of seven times. If you perform it more than seven times, your blood pressure may rise to an unacceptable level, and you will defeat the purpose of this Tao Yin by causing your body to fall out of a natural balance.

Tao Yin and You

As you will experience from continued practice, Tao Yin is a process not only cleansing the body of Chi blockage, but a powerful meditation tool as well. As you become more and more in tune with your body when you perform this exercise, you will come to feel blockage points free up during the techniques. Additionally, you will begin to very consciously experience Chi travel throughout your body, not only making you more virile, but immensely more healthy, too.

chapter five

Jin Guang

Jin Guang means "Golden Light," and is a Chi Kung meditation technique that not only trains your thinking mind to acutely focus, but also invigorates your body with Chi energy while revitalizing your immune system.

Jin Guang Exercise—Part One

To perform Jin Guang, sit either in lotus (cross-legged) posture on the floor or in a chair with your spine erect. Completely close your eyes and naturally observe your breath for a few moments as you calm your mind.

Once you have suitably centered yourself, open your eyes just slightly. Place your focus upon the end of your nose. Then, begin a cycle of eleven natural breaths. Allow these breaths to slowly enter through your nose and exit through your mouth. Do not force these breaths. As each one enters your body through your nose, visualize the golden light of positive Chi energy enter and revitalize all elements of your physical and spiritual being. As each breath exits your body, mentally see all of your negativity, anger, and impurities exiting your body in the form of charcoal-colored smoke.

When you have completed the cycle of eleven natural Chi breaths, close your eyes. Allow your mental focus to encompass your entire being. Feel how revitalized you are after expelling all negativity, while you refresh yourself with the positive force of Chi.

Jin Guang Exercise One—Part Two

After a few moments of mental reflection, again place your visual focus upon the tip of your nose, and perform another cycle of eleven Chi-filled breaths. This time, as you inhale through your nose, feel the golden Chi energy filling your being with positive Chi energy. As you exhale through your mouth, visualize this golden light emanating from your body and encompassing your entire being with positive strength and goodness.

As you practice this Chi Kung, the process of Jin Guang not only permeates your being with positive Chi energy, but it is an ongoing and expansive exercise. You will find that after you have performed Jin Guang for a time, your body will become such a conduit for positive Chi energy that you will be able to extend your positive Chi further and further. It will embrace the room where this technique is practiced, the building where you find yourself, and finally the entire world.

Meditation Remembrance

It is important to remember that Chi Kung meditation is not a selfish practice. It is for this reason that in this elementary technique your eyes remain slightly opened. This way, you achieve a meditative state of awareness while remaining connected to the external world.

Sharing Your Chi

Meditation focuses the mind, thereby refining the energy in each person. This is especially the case with Chi Kung meditation techniques. When you begin to meditate, you should not do it solely as a means to enhance your own physical and mental state of well-being. It is imperative to take the positive energy developed in Chi Kung and share it with the world.

By living your life in this fashion you not only gain meditative insight, but you will continually encounter only the most positive of people and life situations as you consciously add to the overall positive energy of this physical plane of existence.

Jin Guang Exercise—Part Two

In the second segment of Jin Guang, you unite golden spheres of light in two important energy centers within your body. This segment can only be performed after the first part of Jin Guang has been completed because your body must be initially cleared of negative energy—negativity hinders the movement of Chi.

To perform Jin Guang—Part Two, remain seated, close your eyes, breathe calmly and naturally through your nose for a few moments. When you feel that you have become centered, begin the second level of Jin Guang by taking in a deep breath though your nose. Allow the golden Chi energy of this breath to travel to your Dan Tien. Once the in-breath has been completed, witness the Chi energy form a golden ball of Chi light in your Dan Tien. Hold this breath for a few moments longer than natural, allowing this mental image to become clear in your mind.

Embrace the ball of Chi light. Then release this breath of empowerment through your mouth. Allow your lungs to become completely empty as you continue to hold your mental focus upon the golden sphere of light in the Dan Tien. Do not concentrate on the absence of your breath. Instead, see and feel this golden ball of Chi light empowering this sacred bodily location.

When you feel it is time to breathe again, then breathe in through your nose, but mentally see this breath entering your body through your Zuigao, or "Third Eye." With this new in-breath, send the golden light of Chi toward your pineal gland, which is known as the Upper Dan Tien.

The Pineal Gland

The pineal gland is a small organ in the brain, located above the cerebellum and connected to the third ventricle of the brain in all vertebrate animals, including humans. The pineal gland possesses extensive nerve fibers and is highly saturated with blood due to the large number of blood vessels within it. In certain reptiles and amphibians such as lizards, frogs, and some types of fish, the pineal gland is scientifically recognized as the location where the amount and the depth of light are sensed. Thus it is understood to be the third eye of these species. The presence and overall effects of the pineal gland on humans are not completely understood by modern science. It is known that the gland produces the hormone melatonin, and that the gland affects the body's biorhythms and biological clock.

From a metaphysical perspective, the pineal gland has for centuries been understood as a gland that is directly linked to a person's metaphysical "third eye." The third eye is a highly revered bodily location as it links the physical body to the ethereal body via the pineal gland. The third eye is one of the primary locations that one focuses upon during meditation.

At the outset of this Chi Kung exercise, it may be initially difficult for you to know the exact physical placement of your pineal gland. Do not let this concern you. Simply allow the golden Chi-filled breath to enter your body through your third eye and travel to a central placement in your cranium. Witness the Chi as a golden ball of light in this location. Through this practice, the exact site of your pineal gland will eventually present itself and become very obvious, as your Chi energy will be drawn to it.

Once your have visualised this golden ball of light in your pineal gland, and have embraced this Chi-filled third-eye breath for a natural amount of time, then mentally witness the breath exiting your body through your third eye. Feel its power encompassing your body and the area around where you are seated.

Before you take your next breath, mentally observe the golden balls of Chi light existing in your Dan Tien and your pineal gland. See them pulsate with the power of Chi.

When it is time to take your next breath, bring it in through your third eye, allow it to travel first to your pineal gland and then move down through your body linking with your Dan Tien. Feel the power of this Chi breath uniting these two sacred locations and empowering you with universal energy.

Hold this breath for a few moments longer than natural, and then release it. Watch as the golden Chi breath leaves your Dan Tien, passes through your pineal gland, and then exits your body through your third eye.

As with the previous Jin Guang, perform this exercise eleven times, uniting the two spheres of Chi. With each in-breath, witness the golden power of Chi entering your body, leaving you with not only enhanced power, but with sustained overall physical and mental health, too.

When you have concluded the second segment of the Jin Guang exercise, it is important not to jump up immediately, or reconnect with the physical world. Instead, take a few moments to consciously absorb the power of Chi. Embrace the energy before you go out and tackle the world.

chapter six

Yen Chi

Yen Chi translates from the Chinese as "Swallowing the Chi Breath." As is the case with many Chi Kung techniques, Yen Chi activates both the body and mind of the practitioner. With a combination of body and conscious breathing, the practitioner is brought into a mindful harmony of physical and ethereal understanding.

The Importance of Yen Chi

Yen Chi is an elementally important developmental exercise in Chi Kung practice, because it teaches the practitioner the methods of harnessing the Chi emanating from the Dan Tien.

The practice of Yen Chi details that the Chi Kung practitioner brings a Chi-filled breath deeply into their Dan Tien. Then, as it is released, what is known as Nei Chi, "Inner Chi," is harnessed before it is allowed to escape from the body. The student then learns how to hold excess amounts of Chi in the body to be used in times of physical and mental need.

Yen Chi Exercise

You can begin the Yen Chi exercise from wherever you are. In fact, once you have come to master this technique you will be able to use it whenever you need rapid Chi replenishment for physical or mental strength. As is the case with all Chi Kung, it is best to begin by performing Tao Yin to focus your body and mind. The Yen Chi exercise is no different.

When you feel that you are mentally prepared, begin by standing up in a natural posture. Loosen up any tension in your body by performing some light movement. Close your eyes and begin to focus your attention upon your Dan Tien. Watch your natural in-breaths travel from your nose to your Dan Tien, saturating this region with golden Chi light. As your breath travels out of your Dan Tien, see its golden presence illuminating your entire being, as you exhale from your mouth.

Observe this Chi-breathing process for several natural breath cycles. When you begin to experience Chi empowerment, breathe in and hold the breath locked in your Dan Tien for approximately seven seconds. As you begin to release it, watch it travel up to your "Middle Dan Tien" (Zhong Dan Tien) at your solar plexus. At the moment it reaches this region, close your mouth, locking it off. Allow this Chi breath to emanate its power in this region. Mentally see this energy center radiating with Chi.

Your next step will be to swallow this Chi-filled breath back into your Lower Dan Tien. This is achieved by mentally observing the golden Chi-filled energy being held in your Middle Dan Tien. Then, as you swallow, you mentally witness it traveling back to your Lower Dan Tien.

As discussed in Tao Yin (chapter 4), saliva is understood by the Taoists to be "Liquid Jade," a very beneficial bodily element. You are thus causing the Chi you have brought in from the air around you to not be released, but instead redirected back to your Dan Tien through this "Liquid Jade." Once you have mentally witnessed the golden Chi re-enter your Dan Tien, you can release the breath, as now its Chi has been harnessed.

As you begin the practice of Yen Chi, it may only be possible for you to perform this technique only one time. This is fine, as your body will be invigorated with the Chi you have harnessed. As you progress with your Chi Kung understanding, you will develop the ability to bring in and harness as much Chi energy as necessary for any particular action you are about to undertake.

No Savings Account for Chi

It is important to remember that there is no savings account for Chi. Chi is everywhere. As such, it must remain in constant motion. If you attempt to harness Chi for your own selfish reasons, its energy will overpower you.

For this reason, you should only practice Yen Chi when you have a specific physical or mental task to accomplish. Bring the excess Chi into your being, use it, and then allow it to flow free again, stimulating the entire universe.

chapter seven

Pi Chi

Pi Chi, or "Holding your Chi Breath," is the practice of consciously holding Chi-filled breath in your body for a prolonged period of time. By practicing Pi Chi, it is believed that you develop the ability to heal injured areas of your body.

Your Heart and Pi Chi

Pi Chi practice brings you into close harmony with your heart because, as you perform this exercise, you will be monitoring how long you are holding your breath by how many heartbeats have elapsed.

The majority of the world's population is completely out of tune with their hearts. They are certainly aware the heart is present in their bodies, but they only take notice of it when it is beating fast due to excessive physical exertion or coronary disease. The Chi Kung practitioner, on the other hand, realizes that the heart is one of the most essential organs to sustain life. Therefore, through exercises such as Pi Chi, its function is brought into focus, and practitioners maintain a continued awareness of its essential value to life.

The Advanced Nature of Pi Chi

Because Pi Chi involves the conscious retention of the breath, it is an advanced technique of Chi Kung. When a person who is not suitably trained in Chi breath-retention methods attempts to hold his or her breath for an extended period of time, he or she not only causes the natural patterns of the body to be put out of alignment, but also risks unconsciousness from lack of oxygen to the brain. For this reason, Pi Chi should only be practiced in its most elemental form until the Chi Kung practitioner has learned, through experience, to master some of the more subtle levels of Chi breath understanding presented in Tiao Chi and Yen Chi.

The Pi Chi exercise can be performed either standing or seated. Whichever one you choose, remember to keep your spine erect and your body free from unnecessary tension.

Pi Chi Exercise

Enter into a quiet environment, close your eyes, and allow thoughts to leave your mind. Begin to watch your breath naturally traveling into your body through your nose and exiting through your mouth. Witness each natural in-breath traveling to your Dan Tien, illuminating it with golden Chi energy.

After approximately seven natural breath cycles, allow your new in-breath to naturally travel into your Dan Tien. Now, instead of allowing it to naturally leave, consciously close your mouth and tighten up your nasal passageway as it begins to rise. Retain this breath in your Dan Tien.

Begin to witness your heartbeats. Count how many beats go by before you must release your Chi breath and breathe in new life-giving oxygen.

As detailed at the outset, do not attempt to force yourself to hold your breath longer than natural; you are not in any type of competition. Simply take in the breath, and mentally make note of how many heartbeats go by as you hold it. At the beginning stages of this exercise, the average person will count approximately three-to-four heartbeats.

Perform this practice of retaining your breath in your Dan Tien for approximately seven breath cycles. Then release the final breath and breathe naturally for several cycles, bringing your respiration back to a normal rate.

After a few moments of mental centering, begin to focus on any part of your body that may be injured or not well, or simply a location where you may need extra Chi. For example, if you know you will be lifting heavy objects in the very near future, you can focus on your arms.

As you breathe in your next breath, direct it to the location you have isolated in your body. Mentally see the golden light of Chi traveling to that location, illuminating, healing, and giving strength to that region.

As you hold this healing Chi-filled breath, again count your heartbeats. When it is time to release, do so. Immediately bring in a new Chi-filled breath and direct it to that same bodily location.

This stage of the exercise should be performed for up to seven cycles at the beginning of your Pi Chi practice. As you become more proficient with it, you can extend it as you feel necessary.

Location, Location, Location

It is essential that you do not direct Chi at first to your arms, then your ankles, then your back in any single Pi Chi session. This practice will disrupt the focusing of Chi energy to a specific region.

If there are several areas you wish to heal, you should focus on one at a time. Then allow several hours before you address a secondary region. The Chi you focus on for each region will have the opportunity to revitalize the region and its healing energy will not be dissipated by multiple focusing.

Ancient Pi Chi

In ancient times, it was believed that a person must be able to direct their Chi breath to a bodily location and hold it for a minimum of seven heartbeats to affect healing. The longer the retention, the more Chi healing that took place. As the Chi Kung practitioners developed further, it was believed that when they could hold their breath for a total of one-thousand heartbeats, they were approaching immortality.

chapter eight

Nei Tan

Nei Tan, translated literally from the Chinese, means "Inner Cinnabar." Cinnabar is a mercury ore believed by the ancient Taoist alchemists to possess qualities which, when properly harnessed, could lead to one's immortality. The modern Chi Kung practitioner can understand the importance the ancient Taoists placed upon this mineral.

Ancient Nei Tan

In its most ancient understanding, the practice of Nei Tan allowed Taoist alchemists to combine various herbs, minerals, and cinnabar to create a potion they hoped would induce immortality. This mythical elixir was referred as *Chang Shen Pus Su.*

However, at the beginning of the Sung Dynasty (960–1279 CE), the various Taoist schools, having become highly influenced by Buddhism, abandoned the belief that any elixir could provide them with immortality. They re-evaluated their thinking and realized that the road to immortality was only obtainable through highly refined breath control and meditation techniques, which would lead the practitioner to enlightenment. At the point the practitioner reached spiritual realization, they would no longer be bound by the unceasing wheel of cause and effect, known as *Karma,* and would thus become spiritually immortal.

The Practice of Nei Tan

At this historic juncture, the schools that embraced Nei Tan believed that the process to enlightenment began in meditation, where the practitioner must become acutely attuned to their *Ching,* or "Essence." Then, by practicing specific breath control purification techniques, they could become one with their Chi, "Internal Energy." By remaining pure and being one with Chi, the practitioner could advance to breath-control exercises and meditation, eventually transforming their Chi into *Shen,* or "Pure Spirit." With this accomplished, they could then enter into the final stage of self-purification, known as *Lien Shen Fu Hsu,* or "Integrating the Self with the Universe." This final step could only be taken by one who, through advanced purification, returned to the ultimate state of nothingness, known in Chinese as *Wu,* and thus achieving enlightenment and immortality.

Understanding Modern Nei Tan

Nei Tan has evolved into precise Chi-oriented, breath control exercises whereby the Chi Kung practitioner causes Chi to rise up the spine and circulate through his entire body. This process, similar to the practices of Kundalini Yoga, provides the practitioner with not only an enhanced sense of energy and power but stimulates the Chi locked at the base of the spine, thus leading to an overall sense of euphoria. Many believe this stimulated energy is a direct pathway to enlightenment.

Nei Tan Exercise One

Begin the practice of Nei Tan by performing the seven Tao Yin exercises, thereby focusing your mind and stimulating your Nei Chi, or "Inner Chi." Upon the completion of Tao Yin, move into a cross-legged seated position. As is the case with all Chi Kung, the cross-legged lotus posture is best, but if you find this uncomfortable, then you can also sit in a chair with your spine erect.

Once seated, close your eyes and observe your natural breathing process for several minutes. This will allow your internal energy to become accustomed to your seated posture. At the point you are ready to proceed, bring in a deep Chi-filled breath though your nose and mentally guide it to you Dan Tien. Visualize the golden light of Chi energizing your being as you hold this for a few moments. Then release it through your mouth.

Tu Mai

Tu Mai is the Chinese expression that details the ascending pattern of energy that runs vertically up your spine. The Nei Tan exercise directly stimulates this ascending energy. To begin Nei Tan, first place your focus on the base of your spine.

When you are ready, strongly breathe in your next golden Chi breath and mentally direct it to the base of your spine. Hold this initial Nei Tan breath in place for approximately three seconds, experiencing its golden Chi energy vibrating in this bodily location. When you release it, do so by contracting the muscles in the area of your Dan Tien just slightly. This will cause the breath to leave your body more quickly than normal.

A Note on the Dan Tien

As you advance in Chi Kung, you will come to be acutely aware of your Dan Tien. Through time and continued practice, you will begin to naturally contract the muscles surrounding your Dan Tien when you intend to release excess amounts of Chi, or when you are consciously directing Chi to a specific bodily location. In the early stages, this practice must be consciously undertaken. As time progresses, however, it will occur virtually without a thought.

Directing Chi Up Your Spine

With your Dan Tien muscles lightly contracted, mentally witness the golden Chi breath traveling up your spine, coming over the top of your head, and exiting via your nose. When your exhalation is complete, immediately take in another deep Chi-filled breath through your nose and direct it to the base of your spine. Hold it there for three seconds as you did before, and then, with the aid of your stomach muscles, guide it up your spine, over the top of your head, and out through your nose. Immediately upon your complete exhalation, perform the process again.

The basic Nei Tan exercise should be performed for a maximum of seven cycles at the beginning practice stage. If you begin to feel lightheaded before this point, stop immediately.

Nei Tan Exercise Two

At the point you have developed a foundational understanding of Nei Tan, you can move to the advanced level. At this stage you consciously direct your Chi breath to activate specific bodily centers, by causing Chi to transverse your body in a continuous, circular flow.

It is important to note that you must be very conscious as you perform this exercise as it is imperative that you do not let your mental focus slip, or Chi may congregate in one of these bodily locations, where it will ultimately stagnate. For this reason, the novice Chi Kung practitioner should only perform this technique for a maximum of three breath cycles in the early stages. As this is a very advanced form of Chi Kung, you must, through practice, be truly interactive with Chi to truly understand and reap the benefits of this exercise.

The Eight Energy Centers

There are eight energy centers that will be consciously activated in this exercise. They are: *Dan Tien, Hai Di, Wei Lu, Ming Men, Nao Hu, Tein Len Gai, Su Liao,* and *Shen Que.*

The location of your Dan Tien should be well known to you by now. Your Hai Di is located at the base of your groin. Wei Lu is at the base of your spine. Ming Men is located on your spine directly behind your heart. Nao Hu is on your spine at the base of your skull. Tein Len Gai is the crown of your head. Su Liao is the tip of your nose. And finally, Shen Que is located at your navel (see Figure 8.1, "Circulation of the Energy Centers," on the following page).

If you study these bodily locations, it can be easily understood why each is an essential active energy center. Hai Di (the base of your groin) is the center of creation. Wei Lu, at the base of your spine, is the energy center commonly understood to be the location of Kundalini or "the Serpent Power." It is a bodily location where psychic power is based and awaits stimulation. In Chinese it is known as *Zhou Huo* or "Fire Location." Ming Men is located adjacent to your heart. It is the energy center that stimulates this essential organ. Nao Hu, at the base of your skull, also known as the "Jade Pillow," or *Yu Zhen,* is your body's center of harmony with nature—because, if your spine is misaligned, Chi will not be allowed to flow throughout your being unhindered. Tein Len Gai, at the crown of your head, is the source center for knowledge and intelligence. Su Liao, the tip of your nose, is your source point for conscious interaction with Chi, as it is where you physically bring Chi into your body.

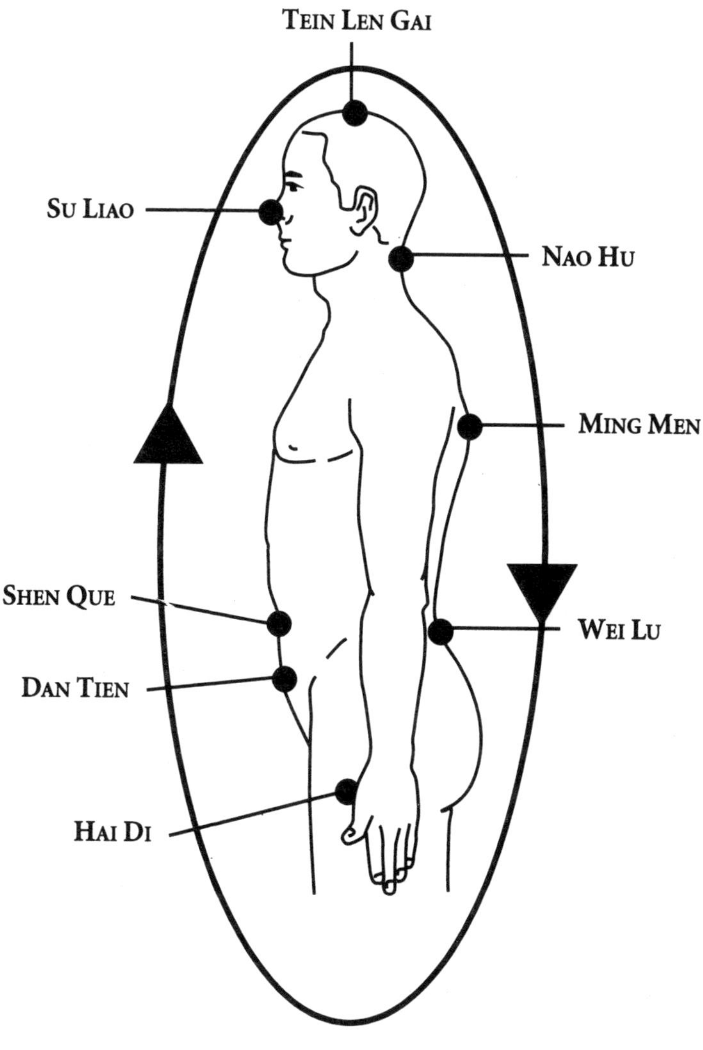

8.1 Circulation of the Energy Centers

Shen Que, your navel, is the location of physical and spiritual nourishment, the source point for your life.

Beginning Nei Tan Three

Now that you understand where your energy should be directed, you can begin this exercise by sitting down in a cross-legged posture and calmly observe a few natural breaths enter and exit your body. When you feel focused, bring in a deep breath through your nose, send it to your Dan Tien and embrace its Chi. Completely release the breath after it has been held for approximately three heartbeats, and consciously encounter the emptiness.

As you prepare to take your next in-breath focus on your Dan Tien. Take your breath through your nose. As you do, witness a circle forming inside of your body, linking all of these energy centers. As your breath comes into your body, mentally see it entering this circular pathway. Witness it flowing in a nonstop fashion, illuminating each energy center as it passes through it. Allow the breath to exit via your mouth.

The process of the breath entering your body through your nose, revitalizing your energy centers, and then exiting your body via your mouth, should be timed to take place in a single, very conscious breath cycle. This advanced practice of exacting Chi Kung may take a little time to become accustomed to. Do not let this discourage you. Through practice, you will come to the point where you can control the intake of your breath to the degree that it passes through the energy centers and exits your body in a highly exacting fashion.

With this mental coordination, you will reach a new plateau in your Chi Kung understanding.

Once the breath has exited your body, embrace the emptiness for seven heartbeats as you witness your energy centers illuminated with power. As with all Chi Kung practices, if the full seven heartbeats is difficult for you, take new breaths in when you feel you can.

The important thing to remember about this practice is that you must activate your energy centers with each in-breath. If you do not, the practice of Nei Tan will not provide results because your breath-oriented consciousness will come in and out of focus.

Nei Tan Exercise Three should be practiced for a maximum of seven complete breath cycles in the beginning. As you become more and more proficient with your breath and energy center interaction, this technique can be performed for as long as you feel appropriate.

The Nei Tan Exercise is a very powerful technique that not only causes vast amounts of new Chi to rapidly infuse your being, but it additionally stimulates Chi that may have remained dormant in your body for some time. For this reason it is essential to remain very conscious while performing this technique. Never attempt to overdo this exercise. Due to the amount of excess oxygen coming into your body, the novice can easily pass out.

chapter nine

Fu Jin Hsiang

Fu Jin Hsiang is the meditative practice of absorbing the Chi energy from the sun into your physical being. It has long been scientifically documented that vegetation receives energy directly from the sun through the process known as photosynthesis. Humans, although not elementally defined by a similar process, nonetheless also draw vitamins and energy from the sun. This is especially the case when we consciously embrace the Chi energy of this life-giving force.

Fu Jin Hsiang Exercise

The ancient Chinese practice of Fu Jin Hsiang shows the practitioner drawing the Chinese character for

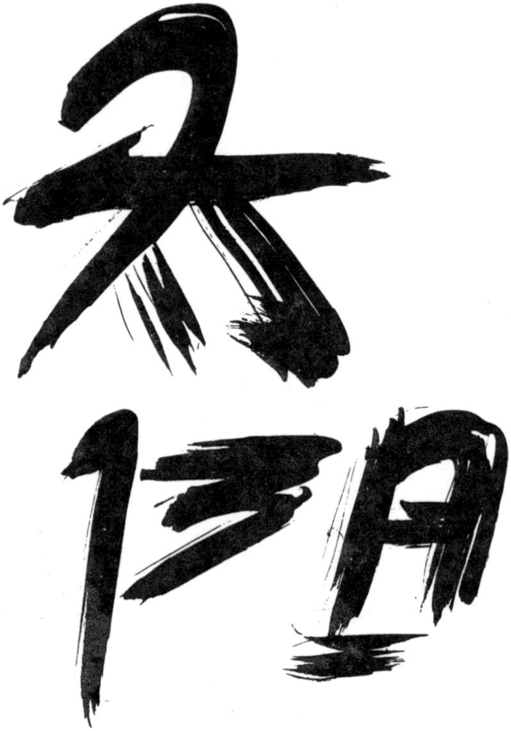

9.1 Chinese characters for Fu Jin Hsiang

the sun (see Figure 9.1, shown above) in a vermillion-colored ink on a rectangular-shaped piece of green rice paper. For the modern practitioner, a simple image of the sun can be drawn on a piece of green paper with red ink. Each morning, the practitioner then rises from sleep, sits facing east on the floor in lotus posture, and places the paper in his left hand. The paper is clutched lightly as the practitioner does the breathing exercise known as "Breath of the Sun."

Breath of the Sun Exercise

To perform the "Breath of the Sun," close your eyes and visualize a distant horizon with the red, orange, and yellow rays of the sun just beginning to crest over the darkened landscape. With your first breath, breathe in deeply as you witness your breath enter through your nose and travel to your Dan Tien in an orange-colored flow of pure Chi energy. When your inhalation is complete, hold the sun Chi breath in your Dan Tien for a moment and then release it.

Take your next in-breath as you mentally watch the sun slowly crest the horizon. Breathe in the sun's energy. Witness it enter your body through the symbol of the sun that you hold in your left hand. Watch this breath travel, in a yellow, Chi-filled flow, from your hand, through your arm, and into your Dan Tien. Hold this breath for some time, embracing its powerful presence. Then exhale through your nose. Witness the yellow Chi-filled energy of the sun radiate throughout your being.

As you continue to breathe in sun Chi, mentally witness the sun slowly rise completely over the horizon, and feel its presence and power engulfing your being. Breathe in this power through your left hand and guide the energy to your Dan Tien. Hold it and then breathe out.

Fu Jin Hsiang should be practiced for up to a half an hour a day. As your sun meditation becomes deeper, you will be able to start with the sun below the horizon and then slowly watch it rise, culminating mid-sky in that half-hour period.

As you continue to practice this technique your being will become empowered with the sun's energy. You will be left feeling full of life, and assured of your fortitude, determination, and ability to overcome any obstacle.

The Sun and You

The mental visualization of the rising sun detailed in Fu Jin Hsiang exercise is the most applicable way for most modern practitioners to take part in this advanced Chi development technique. The ideal method to practicing this exercise, however, is to awaken before the sun rises each morning and perform your Chi meditation in association with the actual sun cresting the horizon.

In either case, it is essential that you truly embrace the Chi power of the sun for this exercise to lead you to an intimate interrelationship with sun Chi.

Sun Chi Meditation

This sun Chi exercise should be practiced as a meditation onto itself and not used in association with other advanced Chi meditation techniques. As in all Chi exercises, you should begin with basic mental focusing techniques. But if you truly desire to be empowered with sun Chi, you should not intermingle this meditation with other highly defined Chi focusing exercises, such as Tao Yin, or your focus will be dissipated and you will fail to achieve noticeable results.

It is for this reason that ancient Taoist monks would choose one Chi-meditation technique and focus solely on it for a lifetime. From this style of highly defined practice, the ancient masters were born—and possessing seemingly superhuman strength.

The Ancient Sun Masters

When the ancient practitioner of Fu Jin Hsiang would eventually achieve conscious interaction with sun Chi, he would then dissolve the piece of rice paper he used for his meditation focus in a bowl of water and drink it—substantiating his connection to sun Chi.

Now, for the modern application of this ancient exercise, once you have advanced to this level, you should very consciously take the paper and place it in an isolated compartment for a period of one year. If you were to simply throw it away, this will immediately dissipate your sun Chi. This is due to the fact that all objects of this universe possess energy. This is especially the case when an object has been used as a focus of meditation.

chapter ten

Lien Chi

Lien Chi (or translated from Chinese, "Melting Chi Breath") is an ancient meditative breathing technique that Chi allows to flow unhindered throughout your entire body. Whereas many Chi breathing exercises guide Chi to a specific region of your body for an exact purpose, Lien Chi does not guide Chi to any specific Meridian, organ, or bodily location. Instead, its practice directs Chi to permeate your entire being—filling you with life-revitalizing energy.

The Development of Lien Chi

Lien Chi was developed in ancient China, and was performed by Taoist sages who dwelt in mountain caves. It was believed that Lien Chi was the pathway to supernatural powers and immortality—a belief based in the fact that from practicing this exercise, the body becomes permeated with Chi. Today this technique is used as a meditative, revitalizing exercise, which not only acutely focuses your mind, but renders your body charged with Chi.

Lien Chi is not an elementary Chi-revitalizing exercise. It is performed only after the practitioner has gained substantial Chi understanding through using Tiao Chi, Yen Chi, and Pi Chi techniques.

Noise and Lien Chi

The Lien Chi exercise is a very exacting form of Chi Kung. As such, when you perform this technique it is essential that you are not distracted by external noises. Because many people live in urban environments, where soothing natural sounds are dramatically overpowered by manmade noises, this can be difficult.

The random sounds of the physical world oftentimes occur loudly and quickly, instantly jarring you from your meditative consciousness. This type of rapid disruptive disturbance may cause your adrenal gland to release adrenaline. Once this occurs, your thinking mind will begin to travel rapidly from one thought to the next. At this point, it takes time to quiet and refocus your mind.

Due to the exacting nature of the Lien Chi exercise, if you are substantially disturbed, it is far better to simply change your focus and enter into contemplative meditation, leaving this exercise for a later time, than to try to regain the interrupted Chi energy experience of Lien Chi.

For these reasons, it may be necessary for you to take measures to ensure that you will not be distracted while practicing this technique. So, while performing Lien Chi, you can use earplugs or place cotton in your ears if you anticipate being distracted by the external world. Though this is certainly not the most beneficial way to perform this exercise, it is essentially important to not have your meditative mindset disturbed by external distractions.

Preparing for Lien Chi

Once you have entered a quiet room and duly prepared for the exercise, remove all of your clothing. You remove your clothing in Lien Chi because, not only does clothing restrict your body, but it also causes sensory perception to occur.

Take a moment right now, as you read this, and feel your body, which is more than likely clothed. No doubt, as you begin to focus, you can feel your clothing.

Throughout much of everyday life the sensation of actually wearing clothing is overpowered by the chaotic world. Once you enter into refined Chi-oriented meditation techniques, however, your senses become acutely turned to your physical being. For this reason, you must take every precaution to not be distracted from focusing on Chi while you practice this exercise.

Performing the Lien Chi Exercise

Once your clothes are removed, perform Tao Yin, focusing your body and mind, as you consciously come into contact with the universal energy of Chi. Once you have completed Tao Yin, and your mind is relatively calm, lie down on your back.

As detailed in chapter 2, the cross-legged Lotus Posture causes Chi to remain "locked" in your upper torso. With Lien Chi, you want Chi to permeate your entire body. For this reason, the lying posture allows Chi to flow throughout your being in the most unhindered pattern possible.

It is important that you do not lie on a bed or a couch. The reason for this is two-fold. First, furniture is generally not firmly supportive, and your spine will have the tendency to relax into an unnatural position. Second, beds and couches are commonly associated with rest and sleep. Thus, not only do they possess the vibration of relaxation, but your mind has been programmed into accepting objects to that end. Therefore lying on the floor is mentally much more beneficial to the practice of Lien Chi. If you have a hardwood or cement floor, lying on a rug or throw carpet will keep you from becoming uncomfortable.

Lien Chi Exercise

Lie down on your back. Naturally extend your arms a few inches away from your torso. Allow your feet to be naturally separated, approximately two feet apart.

Begin by breathing naturally. Watch Chi-filled air enter your body through your nose, providing you with the most essential element to life—oxygen. Upon completion of your initial inhalation, observe as the air naturally leaves your body, through your mouth, leaving you with the sense of divine fulfillment.

Slowly inhale and exhale for several breath cycles. Allow this process to focus your racing mind on the natural process of your breathing. Let go of your thoughts. Witness your mind becoming more and more calm.

When you feel you are substantially focused, consciously bring the next inhalation in through your nose. As you finish the inhalation, swallow, thus, mixing the intake of this Chi-filled breath with "Liquid Jade."

As you now understand, many Chi Kung techniques show you to consciously direct your breath to your Dan Tien. With Lien Chi, however, you allow the breath to permeate your entire being. From this, you provide all elements of your being with positive Chi energy.

As was the case with Pi Chi, as you hold the Lien Chi breath in your body, count your heartbeats. Do not hold it until you are uncomfortable. Instead, release it when you feel it is necessary. As you do so, feel your entire environment becoming filled with positive Chi energy.

In the beginning, the practice of Lien Chi should be performed for a total of seven breath cycles. As you become more and more accustomed to it, you may proceed for as long as you feel comfortable, and as long as your mind remains focused. Many ancient Taoist monks were said to have performed these techniques as their sole source of meditation. Thus, Lien Chi may have taken place for days, weeks, months, or even years in the mountain caves they inhabited.

chapter eleven

Gwar Chi

Gwar Chi means "Extending Chi." This is an exercise where you begin to consciously release the Chi you have brought in and congregated inside of your body. This Chi Kung exercise is best performed directly after the Lien Chi exercise, as your entire body is permeated with Chi. This technique is commonly referred to as "Balloon Chi," as you mentally visualize a balloon in front of your body that you consciously fill with the Chi you are releasing.

Gwar Chi Exercise

Begin the Gwar Chi exercise in either a cross-legged seated posture or a standing position. Begin by taking in a few natural breaths through your nose, embracing its Chi power in your Dan Tien, and then naturally exhaling via your mouth.

By this point in your Chi Kung practice you undoubtedly are very consciously interactive with Chi. Thus, you can readily see it entering and empowering your being. When you feel you are suitably prepared, close your eyes and focus your next in-breath directly to your Dan Tien. Feel it expanding this region with golden light. Hold the breath for a total of seven heartbeats, and then release it through your mouth.

Once your breath has been completely exhaled, experience its power for seven heartbeats, and then bring in your next breath. As you do so, extend your arms as if you are holding a large balloon. As the breath comes into your body, allow it to congregate in your Dan Tien. Hold it for seven heartbeats and then release it. As you do this, visualize the golden Chi energy of this breath traveling up your torso, out your arms, and to the palms of your hands. Mentally visualize a balloon filling with the golden power of Chi that your body is unleashing from your hands. Mentally see the balloon fill to capacity.

Experience this for seven heartbeats, and then take in your next breath, directing it to your Dan Tien. Release it and fill the balloon with golden Chi energy from your hands (see Figures 11.1–11.3, following page).

From this exercise you will initially learn to direct Chi to your hands for any number of situations where you need to

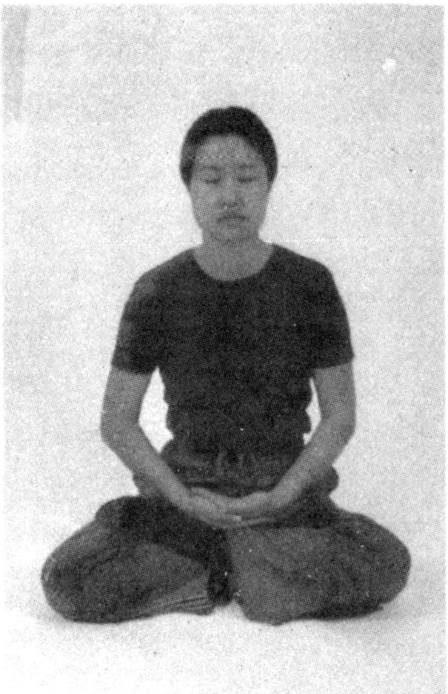
11.1

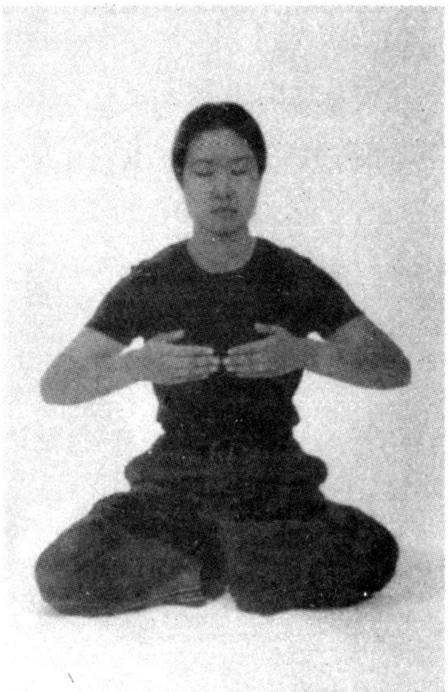
11.2

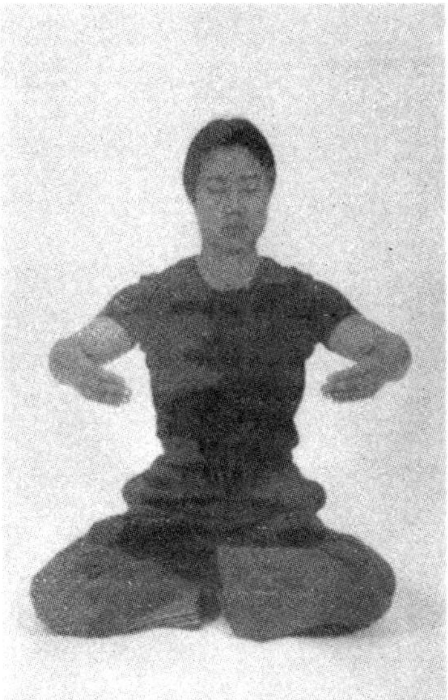
11.3

unleash Chi energy to that part of your body. As you progress with this practice, you will begin to understand that the Chi you have taken in can be directed as necessary to any element of your body where it can be unleashed.

chapter twelve

Yun Chi

The term Yun Chi means "Transporting Chi." This is the stage where, as a Chi Kung practitioner, you are not only able to accurately focus Chi to specific regions of your body, but also successfully extend it from your body.

As you began to experience in the Gwar Chi exercise, you were able to redirect the Chi you brought into your body to a location outside of your physical being (through the imaginary balloon). In Yun Chi, you take this understanding to the next level and actually begin to project Chi from your being.

Yun Chi Exercise One

Move into a seated posture with your legs crossed. Close your eyes and begin to witness the natural process of your breathing. Focus your mind on the fact that Chi energy is coming into your body through your breath and filling you with unlimited, universal energy.

After a few minutes of mental preparation, begin to consciously take in natural breaths and send them to your Dan Tien. As your breath comes in, it embraces your Dan Tien with golden Chi light, but as it leaves its power remains.

After approximately seven natural breath cycles, bring your arms up in front of your body with your fingers pointed upward. Your palms should be facing each other, separated by approximately one foot. Become comfortable in this position as you continue to focus Chi energy into your Dan Tien with each in-breath.

When you feel comfortable, begin to send your exhalations out of your body via your hands. Mentally see golden Chi energy exiting your body from your fingers and your palms, forming a ball of golden Chi energy between your hands.

With your new in-breath, breathe in more Chi energy and direct it toward your Dan Tien. With your next exhalation, slowly bring your hands closer together as the breath leaves your body. You will immediately feel that there is a force emanating between your hands. Practice this technique for several breath cycles, becoming increasingly aware of the power of Chi emanating from your hands (see Figures 12.1–12.3, following page).

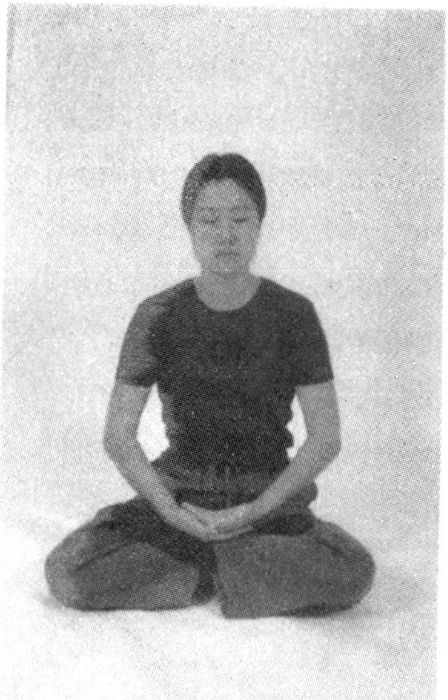

12.1

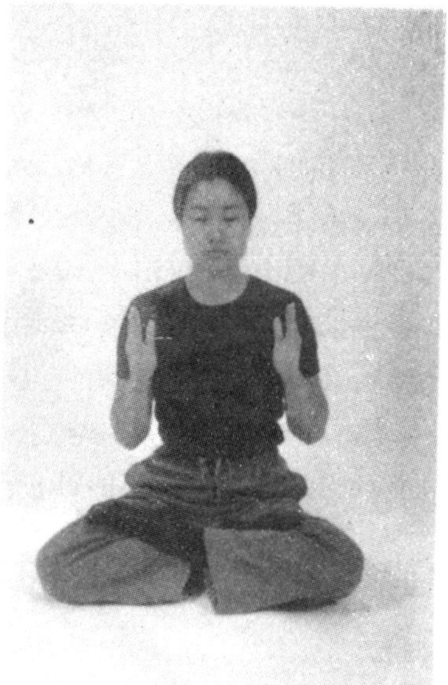

12.2

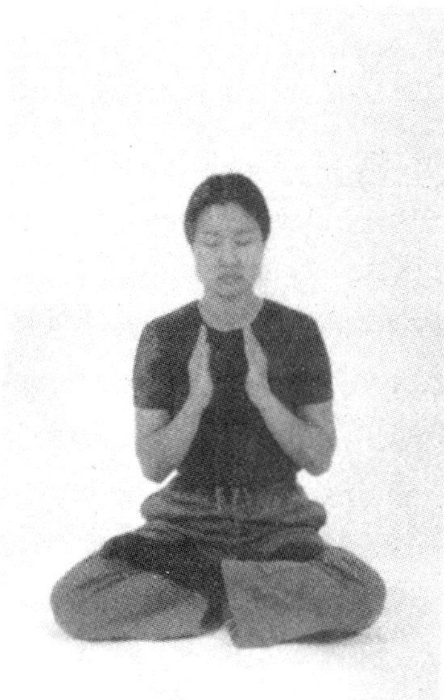

12.3

With this exercise, you will quickly become aware that your hands are, in fact, projecting Chi energy. As you become more and more adept in your Chi Kung practices, you will be able to perform this exercise with little thought or preliminary focus. This is because as you become more and more interactive with Chi, it will be continually emanating from your body. As your hands are direct tools for unleashing Chi energy, several Meridians culminate in them, you will be able to feel the power of Chi pulsating between them whenever you bring them together in this fashion.

Yun Chi Exercise Two

This exercise is commonly referred to as "Pushing the Clouds," *An Yun Shou.* It can be performed from either a standing or seated posture. Settle into your Chi Kung position (either seated or standing), and watch your breath for a few moments as you become mentally focused.

When you feel you are ready, close your eyes and bring your hands up to your chest level, with your palms facing forward. At the point you feel comfortable, usually after several natural breath cycles, very consciously take in a slow Chi-filled breath through your nose. See it entering your body in the form of golden light as it travels to your Dan Tien, illuminating it.

Begin to mentally visualize a white cloud directly in front of you. As you exhale your Chi-filled breath, mentally witness it traveling up your torso, out your arms, and exiting your body via the palms of your hands. As you breathe out, slowly extend your arms as this Chi-filled breath exits via your palms. As your arms extend, see your internal energy pushing back on the cloud, causing it to move away from you.

Once you have completed your exhalation, leave your arms extending, pushing against the cloud, for a few moments. When it is time, breathe in another golden Chi-filled breath, directed to your Dan Tien. As you do, slowly retract your arms to their original position as the cloud moves in closer to you. With inhalation completed, again release it as you push the clouds away from you (see Figures 12.4–12.9, below and page 92).

This technique can be used to push the clouds in whichever direction you feel most appropriate. It trains you to consciously direct Chi to your hands and to send it out through a very refined technique.

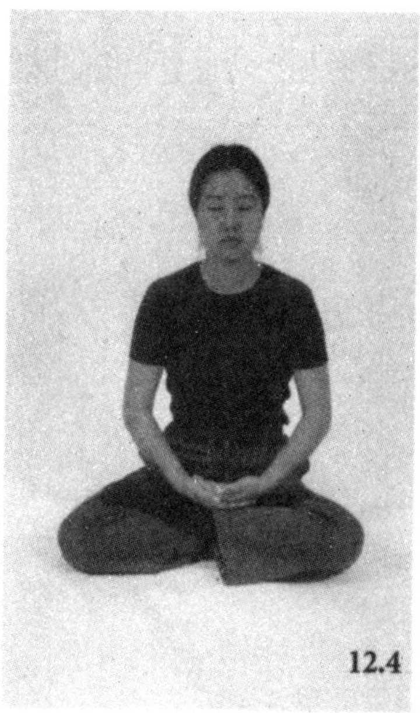

12.4

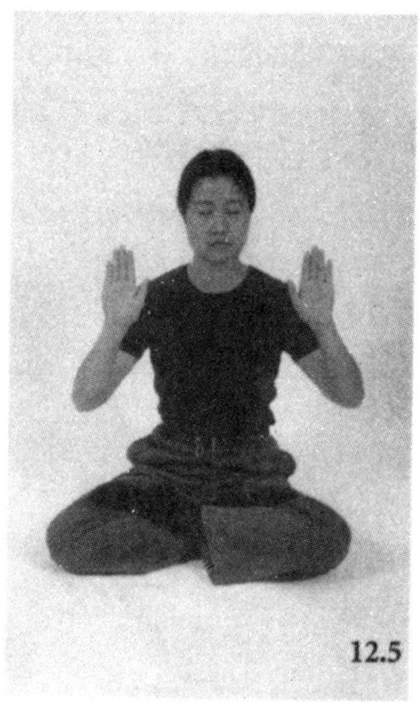

12.5

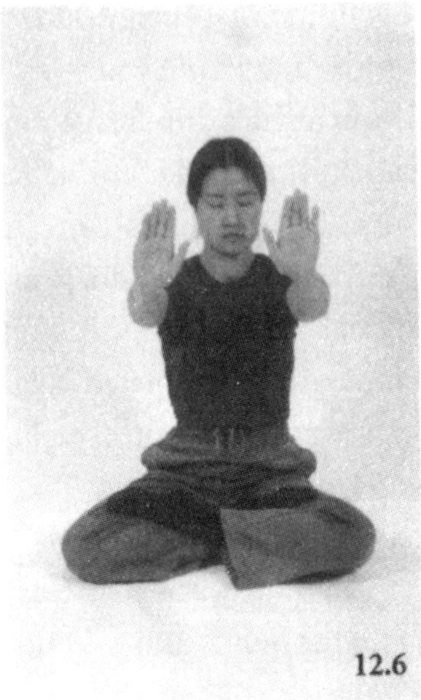

12.6

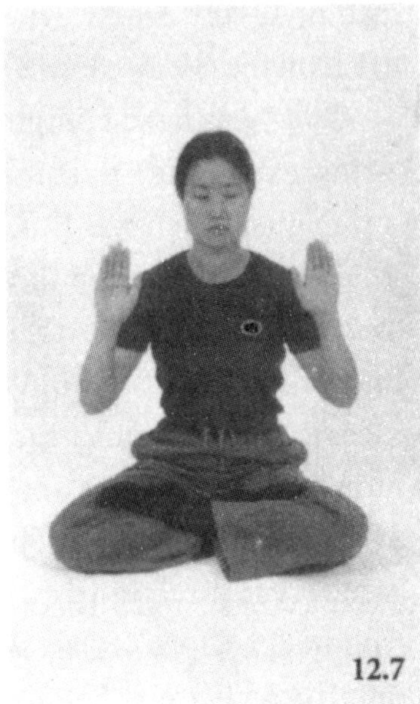

12.7

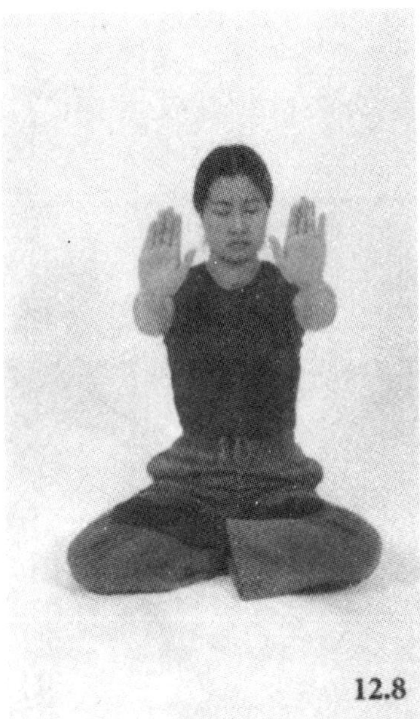

12.8

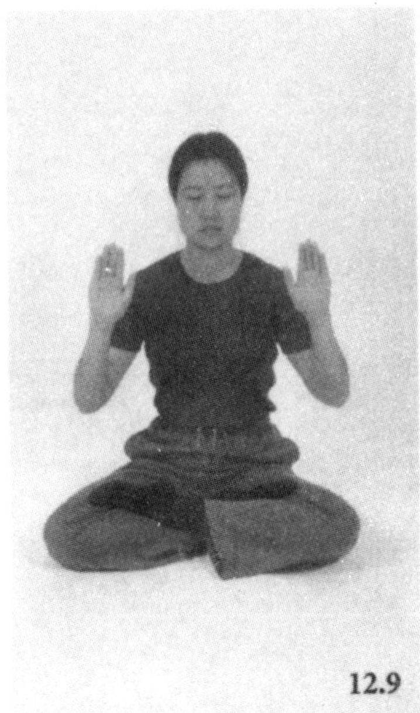

12.9

chapter thirteen

Chi and Physical Movement

Physical movement naturally stimulates the Chi in your body. Physiologically speaking, it is commonly understood that a person who frequently exercises is more healthy physically and mentally. The reasoning for this is twofold. After exercise, your heart beats with increased vigor. Not only does this stimulate this very vital organ, but additional blood is pumped through your veins, as well, thereby nourishing and invigorating all aspects of your physical being. Secondly, it has been scientifically proven that during physical movement biological hormones are released by your brain. These hormones are known to create a more positive mental attitude.

Understanding physical movement in association with overall well-being has been documented in China for centuries. It has long been known that movement naturally stimulates Chi, which causes additional amounts of this universal energy to naturally flow through your Meridians, thereby causing your entire physical and spiritual being to enter into a state of enhanced universal balance and health.

Tai Chi Chaun

The Chinese exercises commonly known as *Tai Chi Chuan* are made up of exacting physical movements believed to stimulate Chi in your body.

Translated from the Chinese, Tai Chi Chaun literally means "Fist of the Supreme," and was developed during the fourteenth century in China. It evolved from the formalized movements of warfare, which monks and soldiers commonly practiced in relation to their various schools of martial arts. Therefore, Tai Chi Chaun is actually a form of the martial arts and was not initially developed as a means of precisely stimulating Chi energy.

From the late seventeenth century forward, this artform has evolved to the level where its techniques are employed in Chi Kung. This has occurred predominately by slowing down the offensive and defensive movements of Tai Chi Chaun to the degree where they have become more a form of "movement meditation" than solely a means of defensive martial arts. Nonetheless, though this is certainly not a negative aspect of the art, it must be understood that Tai Chi

Chaun is still considered an advanced form of self-defense. As such, Chi interactiveness is limited by Tai Chi Chaun's concentration on self-defense movements.

Many modern practitioners believe that martial arts and Chi Kung are in fact elementally the same. Historically, this is not the case. Though these two arts are now oftentimes intermingled, their origin and essence are quite different.

Formulated Chi Kung Movement

In order to gain a more precise understanding of how physical movement consciously stimulates Chi flow through your being, the following are examples of prescribed movements that pick up where the Yun Chi exercise left off, and cause Chi to enter, move through, and be directed out of your body in association with physical movement. From these techniques you will learn how to cause Chi to actively enter your body and be redirected while you are consciously in a state of motion.

Chi Movement Exercise One

Begin by standing with your feet apart, slightly wider than your shoulders. Rest your arms at your side, with your open palms facing your upper legs. Allow your fingers to extend in a relaxed fashion, loosely separated.

Allow yourself a few moments to become comfortable in this position, as you begin to visualize Chi energy naturally entering your body through your nose with each in-breath and extending downward to your Dan Tien.

Seven Heartbeats

During this exercise each of your inhalations, retentions, exhalations, and time between breaths will last for a period of seven heartbeats. This seven-heartbeat formulation was defined by ancient Chi Kung masters as the ideal time for the advancing student to meditatively bring body and mind into harmony as the student becomes acutely focused on the retention and transmission of Chi.

As in all cases of Chi Kung, if this seven-heartbeat time period is too long or you become uncomfortable during the process, then breathe more frequently. If your are going to breathe with a shorter duration, however, do so in a constant pattern in association with your heartbeat; be it every seven beats, five beats, three beats, or two beats.

A natural occurrence of Chi Kung as you advance is that you will be able to extend your breath cycle for more than a seven heart period, if desired. This is due to the fact that as Chi becomes more pervasive of your physical and spiritual being, your body becomes permeated with life-giving Chi. Thus, breath is taken in much more conscious and, thereby, is used much more efficiently by your body.

Breathe and Count

Begin this Chi Kung process of heartbeat counting by consciously focusing your mind on the power of Chi. Breathe in slowly through your nose as you mentally witness your seven heartbeats. As you do so, consciously direct this in-breath to your Dan Tien.

Once your inhalation is complete, hold it for a count of seven heartbeats as the Chi energy radiates from this essential bodily location. Upon the seventh heartbeat, release the breath through your nose as you witness seven beats. Then, expel your Chi-filled breath for a count of seven.

Experience the Count

Before you begin the physical movements of this or any Chi Kung exercise, allow yourself some time to become very accustomed to this meditative, heartbeat-counting process. For many people it takes a substantial amount of time to truly become meditatively focused to the degree where they can consciously experience their heartbeats along with breathing. For this reason, do not force this process. If you do, the benefits of Chi Kung are lost.

It may take several days or longer for you to become accustomed to the initial level of this Chi Kung technique, but it is essential that you do so. There is no need to rush; simply allow yourself to naturally embrace this process before you move further in practice.

Begin to Move with Chi

At the point you have achieved the ability to naturally witness your heartbeats, along with your breath-control techniques, move forward to the physical aspects of this exercise. Begin by drawing in a Chi-filled breath through your nose. Then, slowly raising your arms, bring them up in front of your body, directed by your shoulder muscles. Your palms should be allowed to turn to a downward-facing position, parallel to the ground. Your wrists should not be held in a tight fashion. Instead, they should be allowed to bend slightly as no muscle pressure should be placed upon this part of your body. This initial inhalation and arm-raising process should be achieved slowly, reaching its culmination with the completion of your seventh heartbeat.

After completing your in-breath, and your arms reaching shoulder level, enter into the period of Chi-breath retention, leaving your arms in place as you observe your heart for seven natural beats. As you do so, feel Chi empowering your entire physical and ethereal being, as it congregates and emanates from your Dan Tien.

When this element of the exercise has been completed, slowly exhale through your mouth for seven heartbeats, as you lower your arms downward in front of you. As your arms descend, see golden Chi emanating from your palms and impacting the earth in front of you.

With the completion of the seven-heartbeat exhalation, naturally hold your palms in a downward-facing position as you embrace the emptiness of no breath coming into your being for seven heartbeats. Be aware how you now become interactive with Chi radiating between your body and the ground in front of you (see Figures 13.1–13.5, following page and page 100).

This exercise should be performed for a series of seven complete cycles. With this Chi Kung, not only will you have allowed your body and mind to become meditatively focused, but you will have brought them into conscious

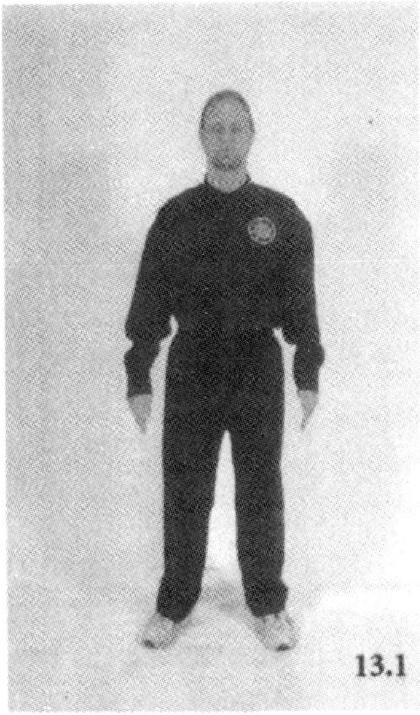

13.1

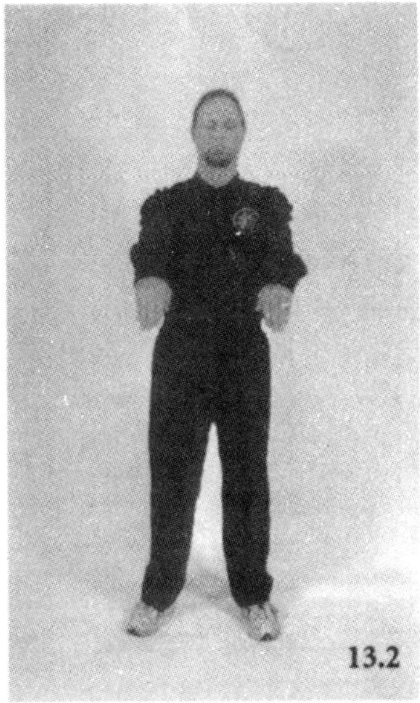

13.2

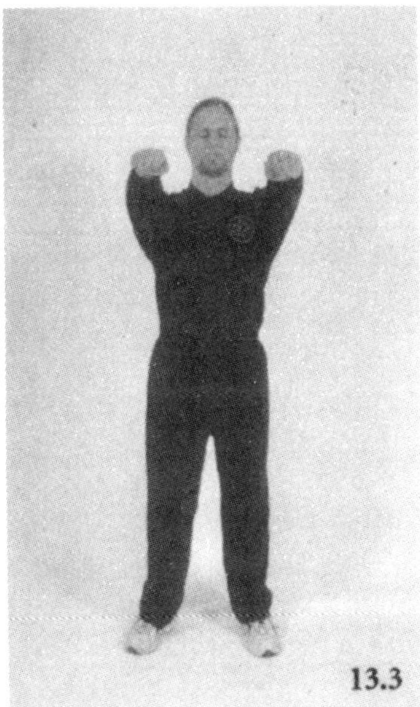

13.3

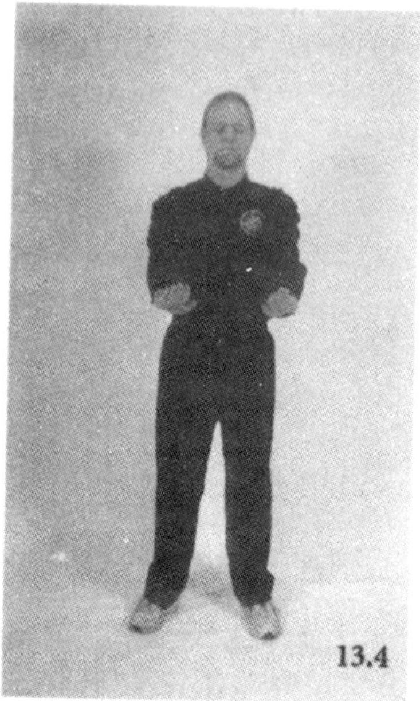

13.4

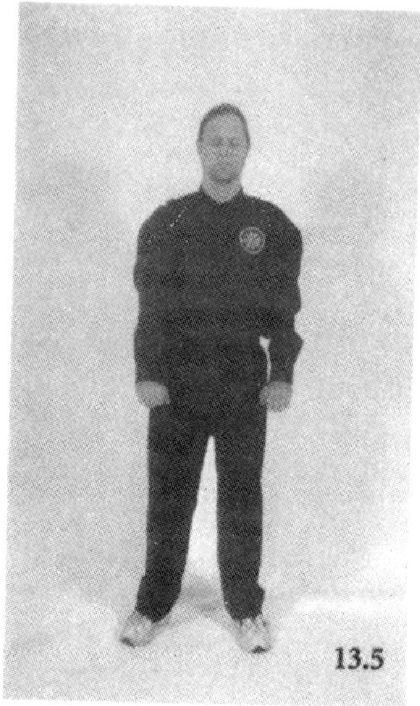

13.5

harmony with your ethereal being. In addition, you will become consciously interactive with the Chi that is launched from your body, directed to a specific physical location (in this case the ground in front of you), and cause it to become naturally reflective (through your being able to mentally see any Chi energy you direct to a specific location reflected back to you).

Energy Attracts Energy

As in all cases, energy attracts energy. This is especially true with Chi. Therefore, as you advance with this exercise you will begin to see how the Chi directed from your palms actually returns to your body, bringing with it additional power and invigoration.

Chi Movement Exercise Two

This Chi Kung exercise is performed in the same seven-heartbeat cycle as with Chi Movement Exercise One. As with the previous exercise, begin by standing with your feet naturally apart, slightly wider than your shoulders. Rest your arms to your side, with your open palms facing your legs. Allow your fingers to extend in a natural and relaxed fashion. Provide yourself a few moments to become meditatively comfortable in this position, as you become interactive with Chi, by focusing on its power, consciously bring it into your body through your breath.

When you feel that you have become interactive with Chi, begin by inhaling a slow, seven-heartbeat breath through your nose and raising your arms from their resting position up in front of your body, with your palms facing toward the ground (as you did in Chi Movement Exercise One). As you do, simultaneously move your legs into what is known as the "Horse Stance."

The Horse Stance

The Horse Stance is achieved by stepping to the side with your right leg, placing your feet several inches outside of your shoulder width. As soon as you are in position, slowly lower your body down by bending your knees. This causes your body to enter into a very firm position.

As you enter the Horse Stance, your arms continue to progress upward. Instead of halting your movement at shoulder level, allowing your hands to flip back, your elbows arch, until your palms are facing toward the sky. This entire physical movement should be orchestrated to culminate with the completion of your seventh heartbeat along with your inhalation.

Leave your arms in place as you hold your Chi-filled breath for seven heartbeats—mentally encountering the power of Chi emanating in your Dan Tien and traveling up your torso and out your arms.

When you have finished a seven-heartbeat cycle, slowly exhale through your mouth as you powerfully push your arms up to the sky, tightening all of the muscles in your arms, upper body, and legs. As you do, mentally witness powerful, golden, Chi energy emanating from your palms, pushing a pure, white cloud above your head. This technique is called "Lifting the Sky."

Dynamic Tension

Commonly known as Dynamic Tension, this physical muscle tightening, used with Chi breath control, invigorates your Meridians with Chi. Thus not only do you develop physical muscle strength, but internal energy as well.

When your exhalation and seven heartbeats have been completed, slowly allow your arms to return to their resting position at your side, as a period of seven heartbeats elapses (see Figures 13.6–13.12, following page and page 104).

You will notice that your heartbeats have increased as you have performed this segment of the exercise. From a physiological standpoint, this is because you have exerted physical energy, stimulating your cardiovascular system.

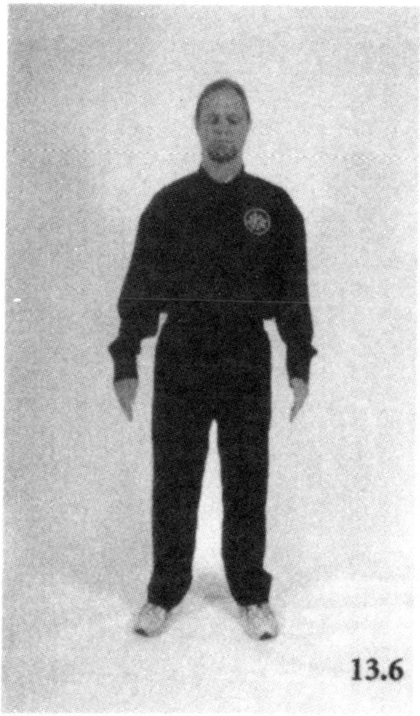

13.6

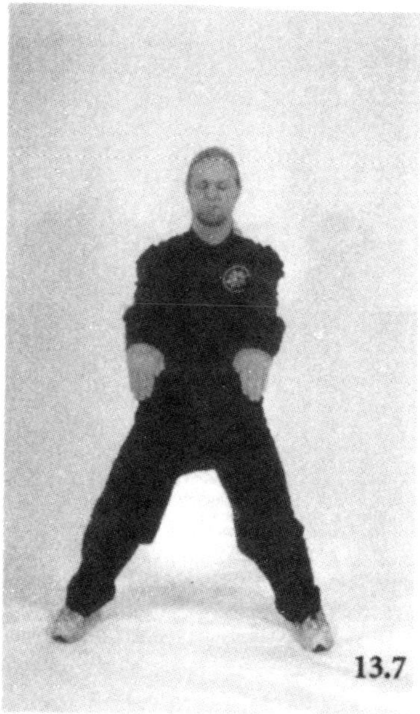

13.7

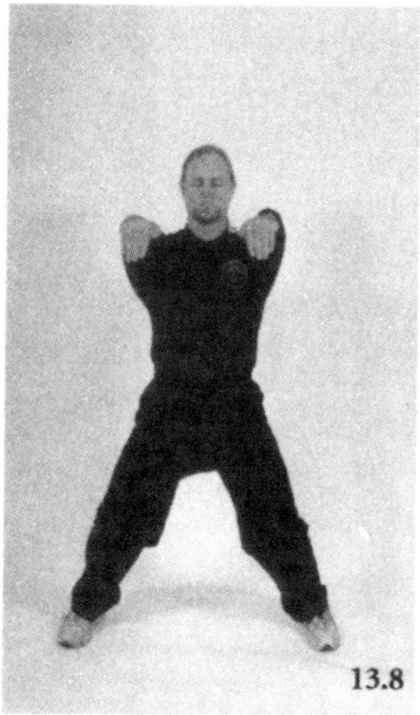

13.8

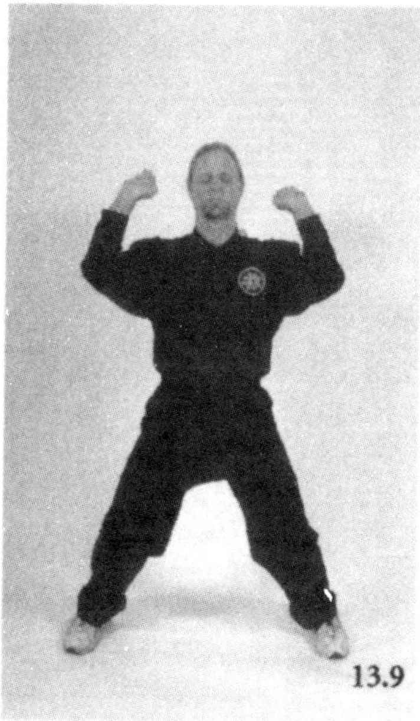

13.9

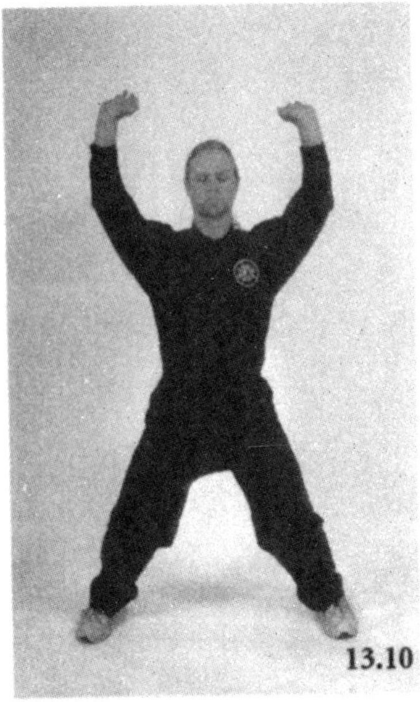

13.10

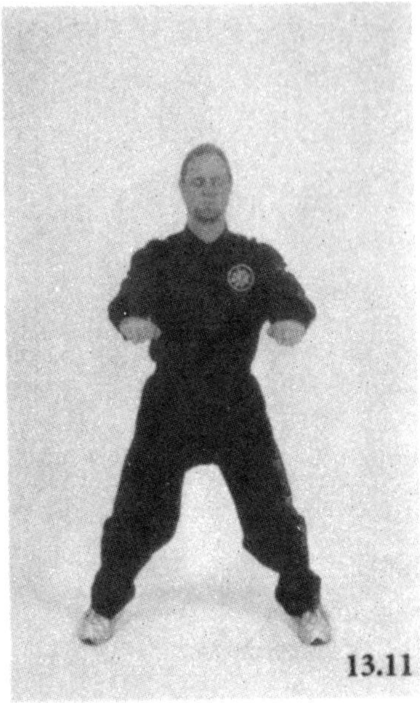

13.11

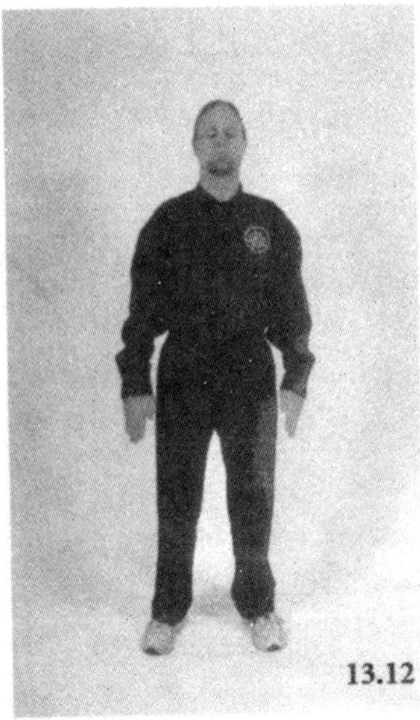

13.12

From a Chi Kung perspective, you have stimulated the Chi flow along your Meridians. Thus both the physical and ethereal element of your being have become nourished.

Allow your hands to rest to your side, and experience Chi-filled emptiness for seven heartbeats. Then perform this exercise again for a total of seven repetitions.

Chi Movement Exercise Three

Begin as you did with the previous two exercises by standing with your feet apart, slightly wider than your shoulders, your arms naturally resting at your side. Always allow yourself several minutes to become consciously interactive with Chi before you proceed with the exercise.

This exercise also uses the seven-heartbeat Chi Kung formula. Therefore, upon the completion of your initial focusing breaths, place your concentration on your heart and begin to breathe in association with the seven beats.

When you have prepared yourself, with your next conscious inhalation of Chi breath through your nose, in a slow natural fashion, step forward with your right leg in a nonformal Front Stance.

The Front Stance

The Front Stance is accomplished by placing your right foot forward, approximately two feet in front of your left leg. Your rear leg remains straight, as your lead leg is allowed to lightly bend at knee-level.

The Chi Hand

Along with this leg movement, raise your right arm until your palm is facing forward and your first finger is pointing directly upward. Your other fingers should be allowed to bend slightly.

As the Large Intestine Meridian culminates in this finger, when you place your hand in this formation it becomes a very powerful Chi-defining tool, commonly referred to as "The Chi Hand."

This inhalation movement process should be coordinated to culminate with your seventh heartbeat. Once you have moved into this position, feel the Chi emanating from your Dan Tien as your body settles into this power-filled position for seven natural heartbeats.

After the seventh beat, exhale through your mouth as you extend your right arm with power and focus, mentally witnessing Chi travel from your Dan Tien, out your arm, and extending out in front of your body from your right palm.

As you did with Chi Movement Exercise Two, your arm, upper body, and leg muscles are tightened as your Chi-empowered arm extends. This movement should reach its completion on your seventh heartbeat.

With the culmination of this phase of the exercise, slowly step forward with your left leg in a Front Stance, as your arms come to a resting position. Embrace the Chi-filled emptiness of a seven heartbeat cycle. When this is completed, move forward, performing the same Chi Kung technique with your left arm (see Figures 13.13–13.19, the following page and continued on page 108).

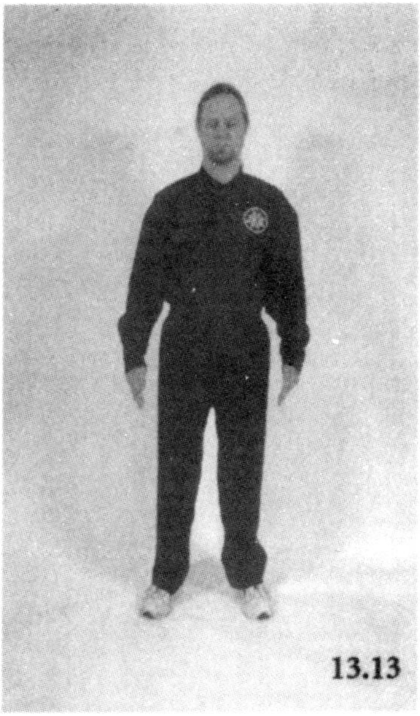
13.13

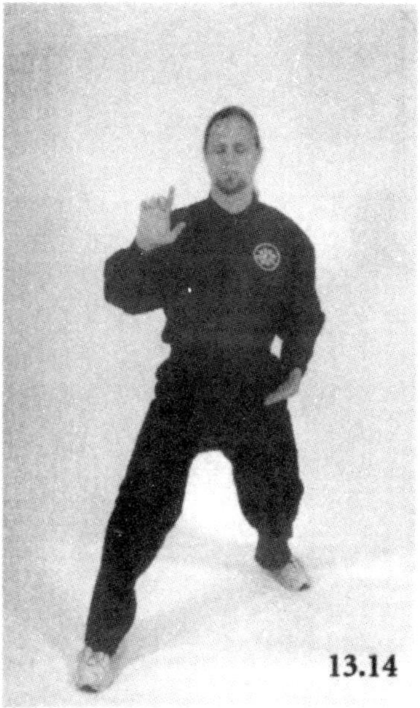
13.14

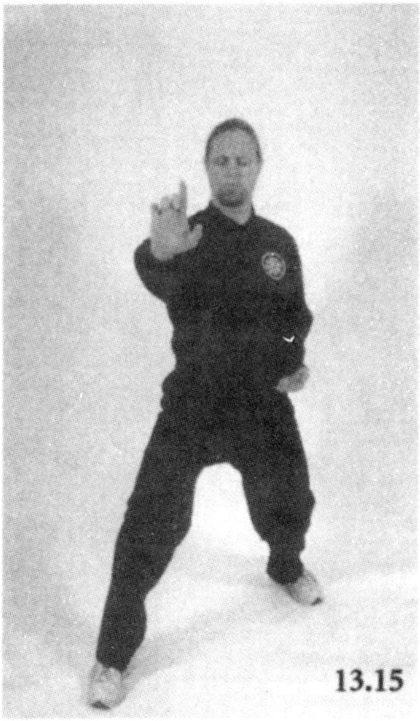
13.15

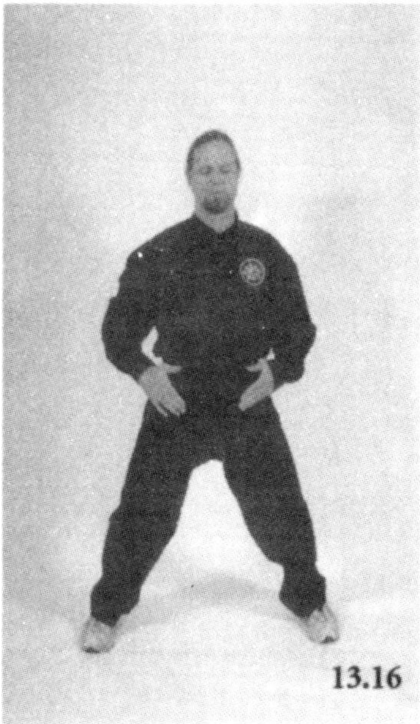
13.16

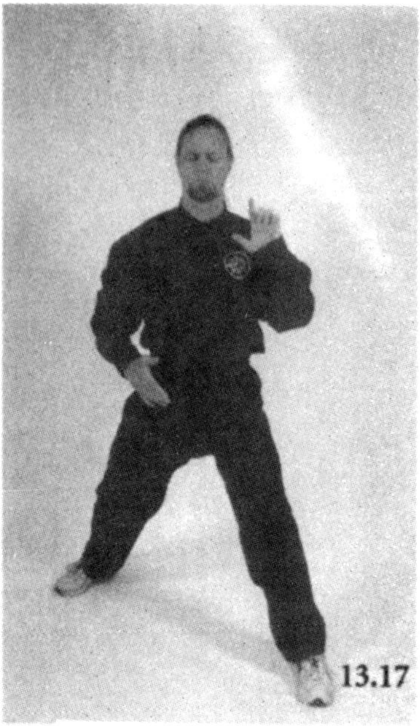

13.17

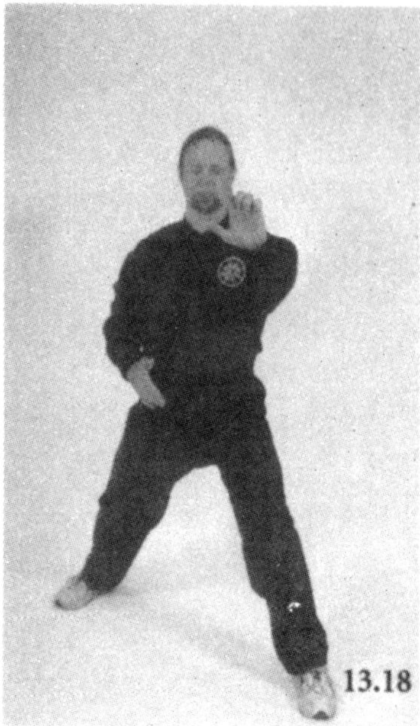

13.18

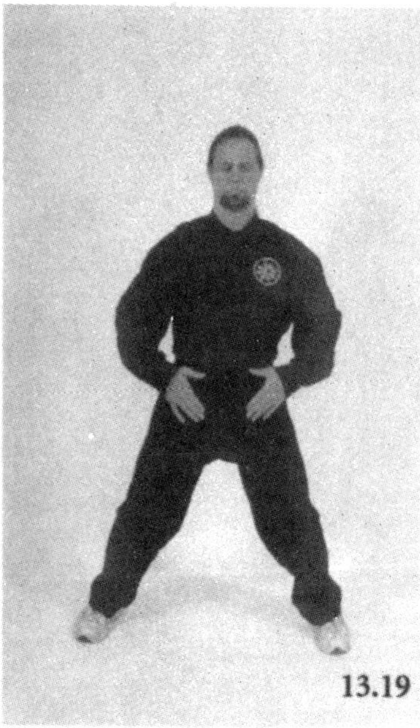

13.19

This Chi-oriented physical movement exercise can be performed up to seven times in order to focus, direct, and empower your body with Chi.

Movement and Chi

It must be ultimately understood that as you progress in Chi Kung and come to understand the interactive movement of universal energy more profoundly, you will realize that any and all physical movement actually stimulates your Chi. This is because of the fact that physical movement causes you to interact with the profound energies of this universe, which, as mentioned previously, are all in a constant state of vibration.

To this end, movement is movement. You should not be afraid to create your own patterns of movement, to become consciously interactive with Chi. Your movement technique can be as simple as standing up and moving your arms slowly from side to side. Even with movement, performed while focusing on Chi will, no doubt, begin to help you understand interactive Chi-movement consciousness.

chapter fourteen

Shou Kung

Shou Kung ("Long-Life Technique") is an exercise that you should perform at the end of all your Chi Kung sessions to not only focus Chi energy into your body, but to also cause it to remain in your Dan Tien in the form of Nei Chi, or "Inner Chi."

Shou Kung Exercise

Enter into a standing posture. Close your eyes and feel the vitality you are experiencing from the Chi Kung techniques you have performed. Feel the revitalizing energy permeating your entire being.

Focus your mind on your Dan Tien. Place your hands loosely in front of it, with your fingers pointing toward one another but not touching. Calmly bring in a breath through your nose. As you do, slowly bring your hands up to approximately chest-level. When it is time to naturally exhale, do so as your palms pivot over, facing the ground. As you breathe out through your mouth, slowly lower your hands to the region of your Dan Tien. With the exhalation complete, turn your hands over, palms facing upward, and perform this practice again.

This Chi Kung exercise should be performed for approximately three-to-seven sessions, or until you feel calm with your new Chi fully embracing your entire physical and spiritual being.

chapter fifteen

Tsao Wong

Translated as "Sitting and Forgetting," *Tsao* refers to the practice of formal seated meditation. *Tsao Wong* is the final stage of Chi Kung. At this point in your practice, Chi flows through your body completely unhindered. You are no longer even concerned with its presence, as it is elementally embraced. With this level of Chi interaction, your focus is placed solely upon seated meditation in order to reach the state of Wu, or "Cosmic Nothingness."

Meditation and You

You do not have to have experienced pure, interactive cosmic consciousness with the universe to begin to meditate. In fact, meditation is one of the most beneficial actions you can perform to lead yourself into this much sought-after consciousness. Through meditation, you train your mind to become quiet to the degree where the advanced understandings of self-knowledge and universal communion may be embraced.

The Nature of Wu

As discussed, Wu, or "Cosmic Nothingness," has been the desired plateau of Chi Kung practitioners throughout history. Wu is an abstract concept to the average person because most people seek only to fulfill their momentary desires, as temporal as they may be. Thus they never attempt to step back and embrace the action of inaction detailed in the Tao Te Ching.

Wu and Desire

When you embrace Wu initially, you consciously let go of your wants and desires. Desires set you apart from enlightenment because they are all encompassing and neverending. How many times have you wanted something or someone with such intensity that you did everything in your power to realize this desired passion? Once you received it, did the fulfillment of that desire answer all of your needs as you thought that it would? Or did it simply move you forward to new and different desires?

In virtually all cases, desire never provides you with any everlasting peace or contentment. Not only does the desire for something set you out of balance with peace, but the obtaining of it does too. As desires never equal inner peace, the Chi Kung practitioner consciously moves beyond this very low level of human consciousness and moves toward Wu. Wu is consciously embraced but never desired. For centuries it has been understood that Wu is most readily encountered behind the veil of meditation.

Wu Shi

Wu Shi is translated as "Five Periods," and symbolizes the stages the Chi Kung practitioner advances through until he or she obtains the level where Wu is experienced:

1. The restless mind;
2. The mind begins to calm;
3. Internal balance and calmness are embraced;
4. The Chi Kung practitioner begins to be able to acutely focus and meditate; and
5. The mind abides in stillness.

Tsao Wong Exercise

Meditation is a mental process where you sit for a prescribed period of time each day and mentally focus your mind upon a specific object. As breathing is the delineating factor to the Chi Kung practitioner, breath should be the focus of your meditation.

Sit in the Lotus Posture in the most peaceful environment you can find. Allow your hands to rest upon your lap,

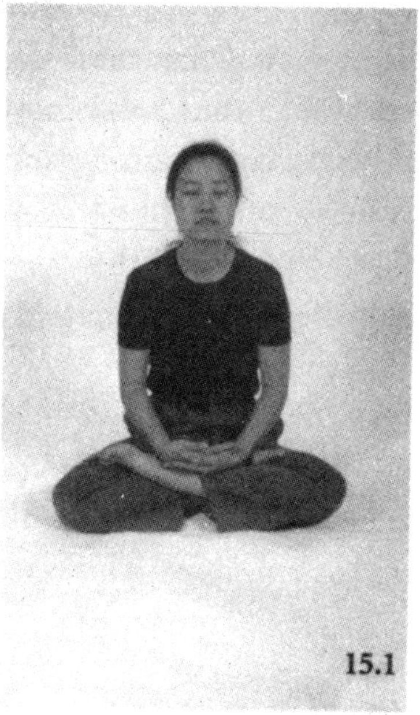

15.1

palms exposed, with your right hand lightly atop your left. Close your eyes. (See Figure 15.1, shown above.)

Begin by simply embracing the initial peacefulness you feel as you consciously sit down, close your eyes, and shut yourself off from the world. Do not attempt to do or think anything, just let yourself be at peace.

After a few moments, become consciously aware of your breath. Simply watch it entering your body, providing you with life, and then naturally exiting your body. Do not attempt to control this process in any way. Simply witness it.

As meditation allows you time to be free from thinking, do not focus on any thoughts. Certainly, we are all trained to think all the time and have, in fact, become very accustomed to this process. But let go of your thoughts. Each time you find yourself thinking about a situation that previously occurred, or a desire you may have, let go of that thought and refocus your attention upon your incoming and outgoing breath. Just watch your breath come in and witness it go out.

Many people become frustrated when they first meditate as their mind is constantly bombarded with thoughts. Do not let this bother you; it is natural, and in time these thoughts will go away through meditative practice. Whenever a thought comes to you, watch it fly away like a beautiful bird on the horizon and, again, refocus your attention on your breathing. Just watch your breath come in and witness it go out. Some people are very surprised that the process of meditation is based on such a simple premise—the witnessing of the incoming and outgoing breath. But this is your key to life—why should you focus on anything else?

An appropriate timeframe for meditation is half an hour in the morning and half an hour at night. In the early stages, however, do not force yourself to sit longer than you feel comfortable—ten or fifteen minutes is fine. After meditating for a time, you can naturally extend this period.

Never force meditation. Simply embrace the peace it provides you.

conclusion

As you progress with your understanding and conscious interaction with Chi, you will realize that not only have you enhanced your own physical and mental conditioning, but you will be empowered with high levels of Chi and have the ability to help other people. Some individuals become protective of these newly acquired skills and are reluctant to share this knowledge with others. With this type of possessive mental attitude, a person commonly throws his own body and mind out of alignment with the natural patterns of the universe. The Chi Kung techniques that once helped him to gain newfound energy and cosmic understanding cause just the opposite, and he is once again plagued by the same Meridian blockages that he had previously eliminated.

For this reason, as you progress further with the enhanced health and personal empowerment that is a byproduct of Chi Kung, it is imperative that you use this newly acquired understanding to help others who have not yet been exposed to these ancient techniques. You will not only enhance the physical, mental, and spiritual health of other human beings, but you will add to the overall positive energy of this planet.

Appendix

The Historical Foundations of Chi

The concept of Chi was born in ancient China, with the indigenous Chinese religious philosophy of Taoism as its central source. Guided by Taoism, and later Buddhism, this science has continually evolved throughout the centuries, directed not only by numerous teachers but various religious and social movements as well.

To help you to understand its evolution, the following are some of the motivating factors and ideologies embraced by the prominent schools and teachers of ancient times, all of which were instrumental in moving this knowledge forward.

The Foundation of Chi

Although there is no exact date as to when the knowledge of Chi was initially embraced, the first text on the subject, *Huang Ti Nei Ching Su Wen* ("The Yellow Emperor's Classic of Internal Medicine") was written during the "Warring States" period of Chinese history (401–223 BCE).

Huang Ti Nei Ching Su Wen

In *Huang Ti Nei Ching Su Wen,* Chi is described as the universal energy that nourishes and sustains all life. The text was written in the form of a dialogue on the subject of healing between Huang-ti, the Yellow Emperor, and his minister, Chi-po.

Huang Ti

Huang-ti was a mythological ruler of China, supposed to have lived from 2697 to 2599 BCE. He is said to have invented most aspects of Chinese culture. Though Chinese folklore claims this text was written during the mythical life of Huang-ti, its creation is historically dated at approximately 300 BCE.

Taoism

Taoism was the primary philosophic system in China at the time when Chi understanding was embraced. Taoism is a mystical school of thought that developed approximately five-thousand-years ago in the state of Ch'u, located in the Yangtze Valley.

Tao refers to "Way"—that is, the way of existing in accordance with nature, internal and external harmony, and universal enlightened consciousness. The understanding of Tao, though varying slightly from school to school, is a highly refined metaphysical method for the individual to leave behind the constrains of worldly consciousness and enter divine harmony with the universe. As Chi is the propelling factor of the universe, the followers of the Tao embraced this science and made the conscious interaction with Chi an integral part of their quest for divine, interactive, universal consciousness.

Lao Tsu

The ancient sage Lao Tsu is credited with providing the first written definition of Taoism, the Tao Te Ching. Though the date of his birth is unknown, his death is believed to have taken place in 604 BCE. The name *Lao Tsu* is translated from the Chinese as "Old Knower."

Lao Tsu is believed to have been the custodian of the Royal Archives in the city of Loyang, the capital of the Chinese state of Ch'u. The primary legend about Lao Tsu states that he became despondent over the continued wars during his lifetime, and decided to renounce civilization and travel to the mountains to live his final days in meditative seclusion. As he was leaving the kingdom, a gatekeeper persuaded him to record his wisdom for the benefit of humanity. This produced the most definitive work of Taoism, the Tao Te Ching.

The second prominent legend propagated in China about Lao Tsu is that once he imparted his knowledge to the gatekeeper he traveled on foot to India, where Siddhartha Guatama, the Sakyamuni Buddha, became his student. To many believers, this explains why the teachings of the Buddha so profoundly resemble those of mystical Taoism, as they embraced the pursuit of cosmic nothingness.

Defining Lao Tsu

Lao Tsu is no doubt the most debated personage of Taoism. It would be unfair to not reveal the quandary over the facts of his existence. Some historians believe the Tao Te Ching was actually created in the third or fourth century BCE by compiling the works of several Taoist philosophers, and was not the work of one single man. Whether this debate will ever be fully answered is yet to be determined. Nonetheless, the Tao Te Ching provided a philosophic basis for understanding that has elementally guided the development of all mystical schools of Chinese thought throughout history.

Tao Te Ching

The Tao Te Ching teaches a way existing in metaphysical nonaction, known by the Chinese term *Wu Wei.* Within its pages it states that action removes one from the ultimate understanding of truth. For this reason, Taoist sages throughout the centuries have left behind worldly life and have journeyed deep into the wilderness to meditatively become one with the universe.

Kung Fu Tsu

Kung Fu Tsu, commonly known as Confucius by the English-speaking world, was the second person to formally lay the foundations of Taoism. Kung Fu Tsu is believed to have been a younger contemporary of Lao Tsu, living from 551 to 479 BCE. Though Kung Fu Tsu's contribution was less dramatic to the overall growth of mystical Taoism, particularly in relation to Chi, his teachings were nonetheless full of magical rites, many based in the understanding of Chi, which could be used to invoke and please Chinese gods. In addition, his philosophy taught that high regard for the state and its royal leaders was elemental to an illuminated life. From feudal Chinese society onward, his writings (known as *Lun Yu,* "Analects of Confucius") have been used to define Chinese statesmanship.

Chuang Tsu

Chuang Tsu (369–286 BCE) was the third individual whose work substantially defined Taoism. Though born into a family of high standing, due to his refusal to serve any ruler, Chuang Tsu is believed to have lived modestly and worked as a minor administrative official in the city of Meng in the Honan Province of China.

Chuang Tsu's written work, *Nan Hua Chen Ching,* is commonly referred to in English as "The Inner Chapters." The work metaphorically details how an individual should mindfully encounter the world. Chuang Tsu took up where

Lao Tsu left off, and detailed an exacting knowledge that "Universal Nothingness," known in Chinese as Wu, must be embraced in order for one to come into contact with enlightened consciousness.

The Chinese term *Chen Jen*, or "Pure Human Being," was assigned to Chuang Tsu because he is understood to have become "One" with the Tao and embraced the illuminated knowledge of true spiritual freedom.

Meng Tsu

Meng Tsu (372–289 BCE), or more commonly known as Mencius, embraced and expounded upon the Confucian doctrines of Taoist understanding. Whereas Chuang Tsu expanded the tenets of the mystical Tao Te Ching and embraced a highly metaphysical approach to life, the philosophy of Meng Tsu was rooted in his belief that humanity was inherently wise and good. His commentaries, based more in a reverence for the state than of cosmic interactions, are left to that of philosophy. As such, he did little to expand the knowledge that each individual should focus their lives upon walking a refined path toward enlightenment, based in interaction with the Tao and Chi. Nonetheless, he was historically a prominent teacher, leading to an ever-evolving societal consciousness that expanded throughout ancient China.

Immortality

The primary goal of the early Taoists was to gain immortality. The Chinese term that describes this state of being is

Chang Sheng Pus Su. To the Taoists who focused their attention solely upon the spiritual understanding of this philosophy, immortality was exemplified by obtaining enlightenment. To the worldly Taoist, however, this pursuit was left to the realms of living forever in order to obtain extensive amounts of wealth and power.

Whatever the motivation, the path to immortality became a highly defined science in ancient China, with the practice of embracing Chi as one of its primary components. It was firmly believed that if an individual could come upon the exact formula for the proper intake of herbs and minerals, in addition to performing exacting Chi Kung rituals and while living a life in accordance with the Tao, immortality could, in fact, be achieved.

Shen Hsien

The ancient Chinese text known as *Shen Hsien* was devoted entirely to the step-by-step method of how humans could obtain immortality. This document, in association with numerous other ancient manuscripts, was unfortunately destroyed by Emperor Chin Shih Huang-ti in the third century CE. Thus the world lost a great manuscript about how the ancient Taoists viewed and practiced Chi Kung.

Wu Hsing

Wu Hsing is translated from the Chinese literally as "Five Movers." This term, however, is more commonly defined in Chinese understanding as "Five Virtues." In English, Wu

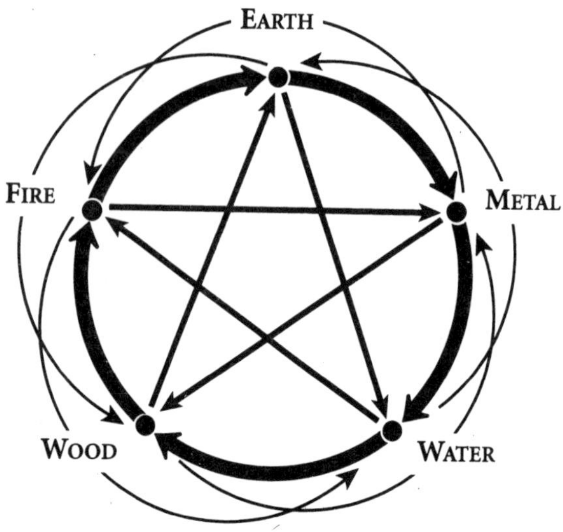

A. Cycle of the Five Elements

Hsing would be better understood as "Five Elements," as this concept details the five primary elements: Water, Fire, Wood, Metal, and Earth, which are believed to determine the course of human existence in this physical world. The Five Elements are a complex understanding of movement and interrelationships. Each element has the potential to give birth to or destroy another. Wood gives birth to Fire, Fire to Earth, Earth to Metal, and Metal to Water. Water annihilated Fire, Fire overcame Metal, Metal overpowered Wood, Wood vanquishes Earth, and Earth destroys Water (See Figure A, above).

These elements, historically understood as the primary components of life, were more than simply aspects of this physical world. They were in fact perceived as metaphysical components that defined the course of humanity.

These Five Elements were additionally defined as possessing a color, direction, and texture. Fire embodied the color red, pointed south, and emanated a bitter taste. Earth was the northern direction, black in color, and possessed the taste of salt. Wood was east, the color green, and held a sour taste. Metal shown west, was white in color, and had a powerful taste. And finally, Water was directed toward the center of the universe, yellow in color, and had a sweet taste.

Each of these Five Elements was also responsible for a specific function of the human body. If a person became sick, it was understood that they were out of alignment with a specific element. The element of Fire was responsible for the heart, the small intestines, and the blood vessels. Water took care of the skeletal structure, the kidneys, the bladder, and the ears. Earth oversaw the stomach, the pancreas, the muscles of the body, and the mouth. Wood was in charge of the gall bladder, the liver, and the eyes. Metal dominated the large intestines, the lungs, and nose. The Five Elements also had specific emotion linked to them: joy was related to Fire, sadness to Metal, fear to Water, worrying to Earth, and anger to Wood.

To the modern person, defining human existence by assigning aspects, believed to be inherent to these Five Elements, may seem strange. From a scientific perspective this may be a correct assumption. It must be understood, however, that more than simply the superficial aspects of Fire, Water, Wood, Earth, and Metal, these Five Elements were seen as possessing intimate metaphysical qualities. For this reason, the people of that ancient time used them as a way of defining the unknown and the yet-discovered aspects of their lives. Thus these Five Elements were a means of placing meaning into a world dominated by a lack of scientific understanding.

Tsou Yen

Tsou Yen (350–270 BCE) is oftentimes credited as the inventor of the Five Element concept. Tsou Yen applied this teaching to all things known to man. He classified Chinese history, geography, people, animals, and vegetables, assigning each a specific component of the Five Elements.

Wu Tao Mi Tao

The ancient sage Chang Tao Ling (34–156 CE) was one of the first proponents of the Common Era to raise the understanding of Chi to new levels of acceptance. He was the founder of *Wu Tao Mi Tao,* literally "Five Pecks of Rice Taoism," a sect more commonly known as "School of the Celestial Masters." It remained in existence until the fifteenth century.

Chang Tao Ling embraced the teaching of the Tao Te Ching and was a healer by trade. He believed, as did many of that time, that illness was caused by evil deeds. Chi Tao Ling cured people by performing magical incantations over them, providing them with talismans and holy water. Each of these remedies were understood to transcend their common physical components and be, in fact, manifestations of positive Chi energy. The charge for his services was five pecks of rice, thus the name of the school.

Yu Chi

Yu Chi (124–197 CE) was another early Common Era master of Chi Kung whose teachings laid the foundation for later schools of Taoist Chi evolution. Legend states that through a miracle, Yu Chi came into possession of the definitive text *Tai Ping Ching Ling Shu,* "Book of Supreme Peace and Purity," in approximately 145 CE. This book became the primary doctrine for many later schools of mystical Taoism.

Yu Chi spent his life as a healer, curing people through Chi manipulation, holy water purification, and herbs. Ironically, he was killed by a family member at the height of his national popularity.

Tai Ping Tao

During the second century CE, Chang Chueh (114–184 CE) founded Tai Ping Tao, "The Way of Supreme Peace" school of Taoism. He based his philosophy on a combination of the *Huang Ti Nei Ching Su Wen* and a loose interpretation of the Tao Te Ching. The primary doctrine for the school was *Yu Chi's Tai Ping Ching Ling Shu,* "Book of Supreme Peace and Purity." The influence of Chang Chueh spread across eight political districts of China, making his school one of the most important religious sects of this period.

Tai Ping Tao initially was embraced by the masses due to Chang Chueh's abilities as a healer. It was his belief that the first step for the ill person to become well was for them to confess their sins, because the mental anguish caused by sinning set the person's Chi out of balance, which was the root of all illness. Once confession was publicly performed, Chang Chueh could then effectively heal the individual through a combination of *Chai,* "Fasting," *Fu Lu,* "Talismans," *Fu Shui,* "Holy water," and Chi manipulation based upon Huang Ti Nei Ching Su Wen.

During Chang Chueh's lifetime, China was not only plagued by disease and famine, but also the heartless rule of the corrupt Han Dynasty (202 BCE–220 CE). Based in no small part on the socio-economic conditions that surrounded him, Chang Chueh taught a method of spirituality whereby his devotees could enter into a meditative state and be released from the pains of the physical world.

Chang Chueh was a formidable figure in the foundation of spiritual Taoism; he was also much more than a simple religious teacher, but was a political activist as well. Chang Chueh formed the proactive political group known as "the Yellow Turbans," *Huang Chin,* and proclaimed himself the "Celestial Duke General." With the guidance of Chang Chueh, the Yellow Turbans set about to overthrow the Han Dynasty. It was Chang Chueh's belief that in the year 184 the Han Dynasty could be toppled, thereby beginning an age of supreme peace. To this end, Chang Chueh organized his followers into a Chinese hierarchical force, with himself and his two brothers, Chang Pao, the Terrestrial

Duke General, and Chang Liang, the People's Duke General, as the leaders. In 184 Chang Chueh lead the Huang Chin rebellion against the Han. The Yellow Turbans were ruthlessly defeated however, and Chang Chueh, his brothers, and most of his disciples were killed.

Chang Liang

One of Chang Chueh's primary foes was Chang Liang (100–187 CE). Chang Liang was a high-level government minister in the Han Cabinet who was deeply rooted in the Kung Fu Tsu ideology of Taoism that proclaimed that divine respect should be afforded to all governmental officials. He sought to destroy any teaching to the commoners, such as those of Chang Chueh's, which were not directly linked to the Confucian Taoism propagated by the Han Dynasty, as he believed that commoners were too lowly to truly understand Taoism and thus should only be allowed to worship those of royal heritage.

In an interesting twist of fate, Chinese history would proclaim Chang Liang as one of the first individuals to obtain spiritual immortality due to his practice of Tao Yin (see chapter 4) and give him the title *Tao Chiao,* "Founder of Religious Taoism."

Cheng-i Tao

Ching-i Tao, or "Way of Right Union," was an important sect of Taoism founded during the second century CE. This school employed talismans, amulets, and precisely drawn magical symbols in order to not only activate Chi but to bring an individual into closer union with divine consciousness.

This sect is considered as a form of religious Taoism and was highly embraced by the superstitious masses of the time period. The practices of Cheng-i Tao have been embraced up to the modern era and have come to define much of the Chinese mindset in relation to use of external objects in order to gain favor from the gods and deities.

Yin Yang Chia

During the third century CE, *Yin Yang Chia*, or the "Yin and Yang Sect," came into prominence as a central focus of philosophic understanding among the Taoist elite. This school adopted the ancient Chinese philosophic concept of Yin and Yang, and taught that the universe arose from the interplay of these two energies, both on the physical and spiritual level.

Yin and Yang

Yin and Yang, literally translated from Chinese means "shade and light." In its most ancient form, Yin and Yang was used to define the fact of whether or not there was sunlight on the fertile mountain slopes where farming took place. Yang was used to denote the mountain slope that faced the sun and Yin to define the slope of the mountain away from the sun. As time progressed in ancient China, the concept of Yin and Yang took on a much more philosophic definition of the polarizing elements of the uni-

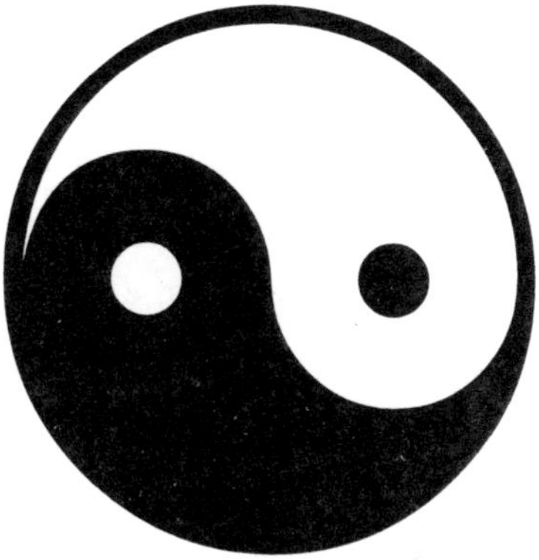

B. Yin and Yang Symbol

verse: white and black, positive and negative, light and heavy, female and male, heaven and earth. (See Figure B, above.)

The first document detailing Yin and Yang occurred in the oracle Chinese text *I Ching,* or "Book of Changes," created in approximately 1100 BCE, during the transition between the Yin and the Chou dynasties. The I Ching was one of the few Chinese texts to survive the burning of all ancient manuscripts that was ordered by the first historical emperor of China, Chin Shih Huang-ti in 213 CE.

As the Han Dynasty (202 BCE–220 CE) came to prominence and the Chinese Empire rose to it pinnacle, Yin Yang Chia began to incorporate the understanding of Wu Hsing ("Five Elements") into its overall teachings.

Chu Lin Chi Hsien

Where the Yin Yang Chia school embraced a relatively sedate philosophic approach to metaphysical involvement with Chi and nature during the third century, *Chu Lin Chi Hsien,* or "Seven Sages of the Bamboo Grove," took a much more radical approach. This group of Taoist holy men not only were talented musicians and artists, but they believed that by the excessive consumption of wine, they could ultimately become one with the universe.

Huang Ting Ching

The third century CE was a period that witnessed vast expansion in the philosophic understanding of the individual and Chi. *Huang Ting Ching,* or "Treatise on the Yellow Hall," is a text written during this period, which describes a Chi Kung understanding whereby the individual will reach immortality.

The text's primary focus is teaching that the breath, as understood to be the primary component of bringing Chi into the human being, must be allowed to flow unhindered through the entire body, as detailed in Chi Kung exercises such as Lien Chi (see chapter 10). From doing this, the practitioner would not only have superhuman energy, but would regain youth, and eventually become immortal.

Hsuan Hsueh

Another school active during the third, and into the fourth, century was *Hsuan Hseuh,* which literally means "Secret

Mystical Teachings." This sect of mystical Taoists combined the teachings of Lao Tsu and Chuang Tsu and blended them with the principles of Kung Fu Tsu's worship of higher deities. This group, due to their blending of philosophies, became known as a Neo-Taoist movement.

One of their primary proponents of this sect was Wang Ti (226–249 CE). He was instrumental in creating *Ching Tan*, or "Pure Conversation," a highly refined method of articulation whereby group members could communicate on the tenets of Taoism in an acutely refined manner.

Throughout history the mystical Taoists believed that Lao Tsu was the highest of all the sages who walked upon the Earth. Wang Ti, on the other hand, taught that Kung Fu Tsu was in fact a higher being and that he was the one who had obtained Wu, or "Cosmic Nothingness," the most sought-after metaphysical state.

Due to the ever-evolving metaphysical consciousness in China at this time, teachings provided by schools such as Hsuan Hseuh began to place more focus upon actively seeking Wu and the "Spiritual Emptiness" provided by meditation. As a result, Buddhism began to be embraced by these Neo-Taoist schools and later came to be commonly integrated with many Taoist sects.

Buddhism

Buddhism was born in India. Siddhartha Guatama (563–483 BCE), a prince from the Northern region of the India subcontinent, left behind his royal lifestyle to become a *Sadhu*, "a wandering practitioner of Yoga." Upon reaching enlightenment and becoming a spiritual teacher, he laid the foundation for the religion that was later to be formulated around his teachings.

As mentioned, legend states that the Chinese sage Lao Tsu may have in fact been a teacher to Siddhartha Guatama, known as the Sakyamuni Buddha, the "enlightened one from the clan of Sakya." This lore however will probably never be historically proven. Nonetheless, due to the similarities between Taoism and Buddhism, and the human quest to enter into a state of divine nothingness and becoming one with the cosmic whole, Buddhism was embraced in China, with varying degrees of success, from the first century of the Common Era onward. During the third century, however, Buddhism firmly took hold in China, and found fertile ground for its evolution.

Buddhabhadra

One of the early Buddhist zealots to journey from India to China and embrace the Chi science of breath control was Buddhabhadra (359–429 CE). Though select Buddhist monks had commonly traveled to China in the early centuries of the Common Era to propagate the understanding of Buddhism, most spent their days lost deeply in meditation and working at the task of translating the Buddhist Scriptures into Chinese. The majority of these early monks were not practitioners of either the ancient yogic methods of breath control, known as *Pranayama*, or in the Chinese, Chi Kung. Buddhabhadra was the exception to this rule.

Buddhabhadra was of the Hinayana sect of Buddhism, and he practiced a style of meditation known as *Dharmatrata Dhyana.* This method of meditation possessed a primary component of breath control. From his refined practices he came to be known throughout China as one possessing supernatural powers. Thus he helped to lay the foundation for the science of Chi embraced by Buddhist practitioners as well as Taoists.

Ta Moo

The legendary Buddhist monk Ta Moo (more commonly known as Bodhidharma) was born in Kanchipuram, India, near modern-day Madras. He renounced his princely status to follow the path of Tantric Buddhism, which embraced enlightenment that came to the zealot through an instantaneous experience of realization.

In 520 CE, Ta Moo was sent to China by his guru, Prajnatara, to relieve the Indian Buddhist monk Bodhiruci and become the abbott of the Shongshan Monastery (also referred to as the Shaolin Temple in the modern era). As Ta Moo belonged to the Sarvastivada Sect of Buddhism, which practiced an approach to Buddhism with the embracing of conscious nothingness at its source, Ta Moo's teachings were readily accepted by the Chinese as they closely parallel the mystical understanding inherent to Taoism.

Upon his arrival at the monastery, Ta Moo found that the monastic life had left the Chinese monks weak and in ill health. To remedy their physical condition, he taught them a series of breath-control exercises based in the yogic understanding of pranayama, which is similar in many ways to the Chinese understanding of Chi Kung. The two primary exercises he is credited with developing are *Yin Jin Jing*, "Muscle and Tendon Changing," and *Hsi Sui Jing*, "Marrow and Brain Cleansing." Many Chi Kung exercises have evolved from these two ancient techniques, particularly the Chi Kung exercise known as Tao Yin, detailed in chapter 4.

The Shaolin Temple

In the modern era much has been written and depicted about the now-infamous Shongshan (Shaolin) Temple. Many would-be historians have dated the inception of the various martial art systems, collectively known as Kung Fu (or more correctly, *Wu Shu*), to the initial teachings of Ta Moo at this monastery. Historically, however, various forms of the martial arts were widely practiced throughout Asia long before the time of Ta Moo.

The Shaolin Temple was commissioned by Emperor Hsiao Wen in the late fifth century. Its name is derived from the surrounding forest of trees that crept up to the walls of the monastery, located in the Honan Province, Tung Feng region, of China. It was constructed to honor the contributions made by Ta Moo's predecessor, Bodhiruci.

As the centuries progressed, the Buddhist teaching propagated by Bodhiruci and Ta Moo at the Shaolin Temple spread across China. Numerous sects sprung from these mystical understandings. Some of the followers directly linked to these teachings held onto the temple's name and constructed new branches in various locations throughout China. This was a source of the continued evolution of Chi knowledge.

As China moved forward into the modern era, the Shaolin Temple became a politically oriented institution, especially during its later years. During this time it was primarily used as a training ground for antigovermental revolutionaries, just prior to and during the Boxer Revolution (1898–1900). The Boxer Revolution witnessed all foreign missionaries and business people driven out of China.

Although the Shaolin Temple was certainly not the only source of Chi Kung and martial-art evolution in China, it has remained a romanticized central focal point due to modern media interpretations.

Tao Hong Jing

Tao Hong Jing (462–547 CE) was a famed healer, advanced herbalist, and an influential Chi Kung master who influenced the further development of Chi understanding. He wrote several books that came to define the mastery of Chi during this time, and helped to evolve the science for centuries to come. Among his works were *Yang Shen Tao Ying Tu*, "The Manual of Heath Preserving Breathing Exercises."

Tao Hong Jing taught that for one to maintain optimum health and possess a constant interaction with Chi, he must meditate daily and focus his attention on Chi entering the body through the breath. He also taught that one should practice sexual abstinence, the result being the body's vital energy would remain intact, causing Chi to circulate more actively.

Tao Hong Jin believed that for one to maintain optimum health and maximum Chi interaction, he must stand with a straight posture and walk with a consciousness of nature and Chi. If one were to become ill, he instructed the person to meditate, focus Chi on the location of the person's ailment, and consciously breathe Chi into this location.

Zhi Yu

As mentioned, Buddhism played an important role in the evolution of Chi Kung in China. The Buddhist monk Zhi Yu lived during the early stages of The Five Dynasty Period (581–979 CE). He was very influential in expanding the interrelationship between meditation and Chi Kung. He devised an exercise known as *Zhi Chaun Fa.* Zhi Chaun Fa lead the practitioner into a deep state of meditation by having the practitioner focus attention on the breath. It was designed to then systematically free the practitioner from desire by focusing Chi on the six physical centers of desire.

These bodily locations are more commonly known as the *chakras.* There are normally seven chakras detailed. Zhi Yu did not recognize the seventh chakra, located on the crown of the head, however, as no desire is held in this energy center, which is also the bodily location where cosmic consciousness may be encountered.

By first obtaining a deep state of meditation, and then focusing Chi on the centers of desire, Zhi Yu taught that desire was literally burned out of the practitioner through the positive power of Chi.

Zim Chueng Shen

Zim Chueng Shen was a Chi Kung master who lived during the early part of the Tang Dynasty (618–906 CE). He taught that eating meat was adverse not only to a person's health, but to his or her conscious interaction with Chi as well. He based his premise on the fact that all elements of this universe, both animate and inanimate, are alive and thriving with Chi. If you take the life of an animal and cause its Chi to stop flowing, then you have altered the natural balance of the universe. If you then go on to eat the animal, you are consuming a very negative form of Chi, which will not only affect your later interaction with Chi, but will cause you to become prone to illness due to ingesting a substance with nonactive Chi.

Zim Chueng Shen taught five steps to obtain conscious Chi interaction:

1. Observe your body as a sacred vessel. Do not eat meat and drink wine.
2. Find a solitary place and practice Chi Kung daily.
3. Meditate. Stop thinking, seeking new experiences, and storing thoughts, for they will cause you nothing but grief.
4. Sit and forget. Forget both you and me. Forget heaven and earth. Forget all things.
5. All things can be known if you touch the source of Chi. You can control Yin and Yang, and exist in the everlasting universe.

Zim Chueng Shen wrote many texts on Chi Kung and meditation. Perhaps his most profound work was titled *Zhou Wang Lun,* "Sitting and Forgetting."

Lung Dong Bin

Lung Dong Bin was one of the most influential teachers of Chi Kung during the early Tang Dynasty. He wrote *Bai Zui Bei,* "The One-Hundred-Word Epitaph." In this one-hundred-word manuscript, he poetically states that one should refrain from doing anything that is not absolutely necessary. That every movement should possess a reason, and that all you should do with your life is stop speaking, meditate, and encounter Chi.

Wu Tsung

Emperor Wu Tsung (814–850 CE) was one of the key foes of the proliferation of Buddhism throughout China during the Tang Dynasty. During this dynasty, the China empire was the largest and most wealthiest on Earth. Arts and philosophy flourished and the knowledge of Chi was highly embraced.

Wu Tsung was a staunch supporter of Taoism. As such, he saw to it that many of the Buddhist temples located in China were destroyed and many of its adherents put to death, thus demonstrating how the philosophic inclinations of a political leader could truly affect the evolution of religion. From the acts of Wu Tsung, many of the Buddhist-oriented, Chi development teachings were left to monks who went into hiding in mountain caves, and practiced their techniques in secret.

Yun Chi-Chi Chien

Yun Chi-Chi Chien, "The Cloud Book and Seven Strips of Bamboo," is one of the most important canons composed on the subject of Chi Kung. Written in the eleventh century, it details all of the known exercises of Taoist Chi Kung through the Song Dynasty (960–1279 CE). In addition, it details biographies and medical practices common to the Chinese foundations of Chi.

Tai-i Tao

Hsiao Pao Chen was the founder of the *Tai-i Tao,* "Way of the Supreme Tao" school of Taoism. Though the school was a sect of metaphysical Taoism, it possessed much reverence for the works of Kung Fu Tsu, thus bridging the gap between religious and political Taoism.

Hsiao Pao Chen found much of his inspiration from the *Cheng-i Tao,* "Way of Just Unity" school of Taoism. Hsiano's disciples were active participants of *Fu Lu Pai,* "Magical or Alchemistic Taoism."

The primary deity this school worshiped was *Huang Lao Chun,* "Ancient Yellow Lord," who was believed to have descended to Earth several times to help mankind. Lao Tsu was believed to be one of his incarnations.

Tai-i Tao was a strictly monastic sect of Taoism. Its followers believed that one could not achieve the higher realms of consciousness or immortality if they were burdened by the demands of society. Thus they retreated to monasteries to heighten their meditative and Chi awareness and hone their alchemistic skills. The sect fell into decline during the Yuan Dynasty (1279–1368 CE).

Tai-i Chin Hua Tsung Chih

Tai-i Chin Hua Tsung Chih, or "The Golden Flower of the Supreme One," is a seventeenth-century text detailing highly exact techniques of Chi Kung and meditation. It teaches that the inner light of Chi can be trained to consciously circulate in your body, thus creating the "Golden Flower"—a symbolic term describing your pure inner spirit merging with the cosmic whole, and creating a divine union.

Chi in the Modern Era

As the centuries progressed, the science of Chi was passed on and advanced not only within China, but in Korea and Japan, too. The techniques of Chi Kung, once believed only mastered by monks and holy men, have evolved to the state where today this ancient knowledge can be accessed by anyone who takes the time to consciously come into an interactive relationship with this universal energy.

Glossary

Bodhidharma: Indian monk who traveled to China in 520 CE and became the abbott of the Shaolin monastery.

Buddhabhadra (359–429): Indian Buddhist monk who traveled to China.

Chang Chueh (114–184 CE): Founder of Tai Ping Tao, "Way of Supreme Peace school."

Chang Liang (100–187 CE): Chinese statesman.

Chang Sheng Pus Su: Metaphysical immortality.

Chang Tao Ling (34–156 CE): Founder of the "Five Pecks of Rice" school of Taoism.

Chen Jen: Pure Human Being.

Chi Kung: Method of consciously bring Universal Energy into the human body.

Chi: Universal Energy.

Ching Kung: Passive Chi Kung techniques.

Ching-i Tao: Way of Right Union School, second-century CE.

Chi-po: The minister of Huang-ti.

Chu Lin Chi Hsien: Seven Sages of the Bamboo Grove, third century CE Taoist sect.

Ch'u: Chinese State located in the Yangtze Valley.

Chuang Tsu (369–286 BCE): Chinese philosopher. Author of *The Inner Chapters.*

Da Chang Jing: Large Intestine Meridian.

Dan Jing: Gall Bladder Meridian.

Dan Tien: Field of Elixir.

Fan Hu Zi: Reverse Breathing Chu Kung technique.

Fei Jing: Lung Meridian.

Fu Jin Hsiang: Meditative practice of absorbing Chi from the sun.

Fu Lu: Talismans.

Fu Shui: Holy water.

Gan Jing: Liver Meridian.

Gwar Chi: Extending Chi.

Hsiao Pao Chen: Third-century founder of Tai-i Tao.

Hsuan Hseuh: Secret Mystical Teachings. Third century CE sect of mystical Taoists.

Huang Ti Nei Ching Su Wen: *The Yellow Emperor's Classic of Internal Medicine.*

Huang-ti: The Yellow Emperor.

I Ching: *Book of Changes.*

Jin Guang: Golden Light.

Jing: Meridians.

Kou Ch'ih: Chattering of the Teeth.

Kung Fu Tsu: Chinese statesman and philosopher. More commonly known as Confucius.

Lao Tsu: Chinese philosopher. Author of the *Tao Te Ching.*

Lien Chi: Melting Chi breath.

Lun Yu: The Analects of Confucius.

Lung Dong Bin: Seventh-century Chi Kung master.

Meng Tsu (372–289 BCE): Chinese philospher, more commonly known as Mencius.

Nan Hua Chen Ching: The Inner Chapters.

Nei Chi: Internal Chi.

Nei Tan: Inner Cinnabar.

Pang Guang Jing: Bladder Meridian.

Pi Chi: Holding your Chi Breath.

Pi Jing: Spleen Meridian.

Sao Jian Jing: Triple Warmer Meridian.

Shen Hsien: Third-century Taoist text detailing the method to immortality.

Shou Kung: Long-Life Technique.

Shun Jing: Kidney Meridian.

Siddhartha Guatama (563–483 BCE): The Buddha.

Tai Chi Chaun: Fist of the Supreme.

Tai Ping Ching Ling Shu: *Book of Supreme Peace and Purity.*

Tai Ping Tao: The Way of Supreme Peace school of Taoism.

Tai-i Chin Hua Tsung Chih: *The Golden Flower of the Supreme One.* Seventeenth-century text on Chi Kung.

Tai-i Tao: Way of the Supreme Tao. Thirteenth-century Taoist sect.

Tao Hong Jing (462–547 CE): Taoist healer.

Tao Te Ching: The book that describes mystical Taoism.

Tao Yin: Stretching and Contracting the Body.

Tao: The Way.

Tiao Chi: The Harmonizing of the Breath.

Tsao Wong: Sitting and Forgetting.

Tsou Yen (350–270 BCE): Inventor of the Five Element understanding.

Tun To: Chi Kung technique of consciously swallowing saliva.

Tung Kung: Active style of Chi Kung.

Wai Chi: Outer Chi.

Wang Ti (226–249 CE): Taoist master.

Wei Jing: Stomach Meridian.

Wu Hsing: Five Movers or Five Virtues.

Wu Shi: Five Periods.

Wu Tao Mi Tao: Five Pecks of Rice Taoism.

Wu Tsang: The Five Organs.

Wu Tsung (814–850 CE): Chinese emperor.

Wu Wei: Nonaction.

Wu: Cosmic Nothingness.

Xian Chang Jing: Small Intestine Meridian.

Xin Bao Jing: Heart Constrictor Meridian.

Xin Jing: Heart Meridian.

Yen Chi: Swallowing the Chi Breath.

Yin and Yang: Shade and Light.

Yin Yang Chia: School of Yin and Yang.

Yu Chi (124–197 CE): Taoist master.

Yu Chiang: Saliva.

Yun Chi: *(Chi Chien) The Cloud Book and Seven Strips of Bamboo.* Eleventh-century text on Chi Kung.

Yun Chi: Transporting Chi.

Zhen Hu Zi: Normal Breathing Chi Kung technique.

Zim Chueng Shen: Seventh-century Chi Kung master.

Suggested Reading

Campany, Robert Ford. *To Live as Long as Heaven and Earth: A Translation and Study of Ge Hong's Tradition of Divine Transcendence.* Berkeley: University of California Press, 2002.

Davis, Edward L. *Society and the Supernatural in Song China.* Honolulu: University of Hawaii Press, 2001.

Ebrey, Patricia Buckley. *Chinese Civilization: A Sourcebook.* New York: Free Press, 1993.

———. *The Cambridge Illustrated History of China.* Cambridge: Cambridge University Press, 1999.

Fisher-Schreiber, Ingrid, and David O'Neal, eds. Translated by Werner Wunsche. *The Shambhala Dictionary of Taoism.* Boston: Shambhala Publications, 1996.

Gernet, Jacques. *A History of Chinese Civilization.* Cambridge: Cambridge University Press, 1985.

Huang, Xiankuan. *Chinese Qigong Acupressure Therapy: A Traditional Healing Technology for the Modern World.* Bejing: Foreign Language Press, 2000.

Hymes, Robert. *Way and Byway: Taoism, Local Religion, and Models of Divinity in Sung and Modern China.* Berkeley: University of California Press, 2002.

Kohn, Livia, and Harold D. Roth, ed. *Daoist Identity.* Honolulu: University of Hawaii Press, 2002.

Paludan, Ann, and Toby Wilkinson. *Chronicle of the Chinese Emperors: The Reign-By-Reign Record of the Rulers of Imperial China.* London: Thames & Hudson, 1998.

Pas, Julian F., and Man Kam Leung. *Historical Dictionary of Taoism.* Landham: Scarecrow Press, 1998.

Pines, Yuri. *Foundations of Confucian Thought: Intellectual Life in the Chunqiu Period, 722–453* BCE. Honolulu: University of Hawaii Press, 2001.

Roberts, J. A. G. *A Concise History of China.* Cambridge: Harvard University Press, 1999.

Sharf, Robert H. *Coming to Terms with Chinese Buddhism: A Reading of the Treasure Store Treatis.* Honolulu: University of Hawaii Press, 2001.

Shou-Yu Liang, Wu and Wen-Ching. *Qigong Empowerment: A Guide to Medical, Taoist, Buddhist, Wushu Energy Cultivation.* East Providence: Way of the Dragon, 1996.

Strickmann, Michel, and Bernard Faure, eds. *Chinese Magical Medicine.* Stanford: Stanford University Press, 2002.

Tzu, Shui-Ch'Ing, ed., *Cultivating Stillness: A Taoist Manual for Transforming Body and Mind.* Boston: Shambhala Publications, 1992.

Wong, Eva, trans. *Harmonizing Yin & Yang.* Boston: Shambhala Publications, 1997.

———. *Teachings of the Tao: Readings from the Taoist Spiritual Tradition.* Boston: Shambhala Publications, 1997.

———, trans. *The Shambhala Guide to Taoism.* Boston: Shambhala Publications, 1997.

———, trans. *The Tao of Health, Longevity, and Immortality: The Teachings of Immortals Chung and Lu.* Boston: Shambhala Publications, 1997.

Yang, Jwing-Ming. *The Root of Chinese Qigong: Secrets for Health, Longevity & Enlightenment.* Boston: YMAA Publications.

Index

BOOKS OF RELATED INTEREST

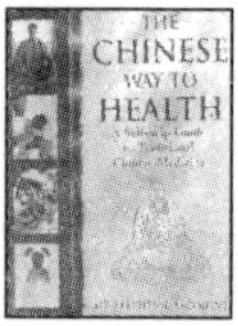

THE CHINESE WAY TO HEALTH

A Self-help Guide to Traditional Chinese Medicine

Dr. Stephen Gascoigne

ISBN: 81-7822-160-8

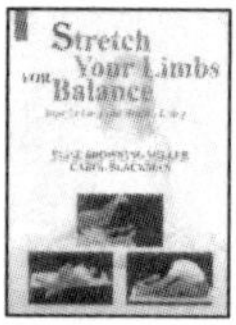

STRETCH YOUR LIMBS FOR BALANCE

Yoga for Long and Healthy Living

Elise Browning Miller
Carol Blackman

ISBN: 81-7822-132-2

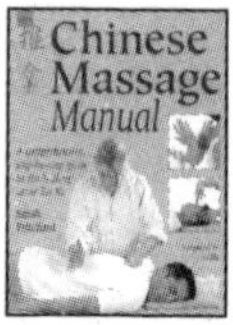

CHINESE MASSAGE MANUAL

A Comprehensive, Step-by-Step Guide to the Healing Art of Tui Na

Sarah Pritchard

ISBN: 81-7822-122-5

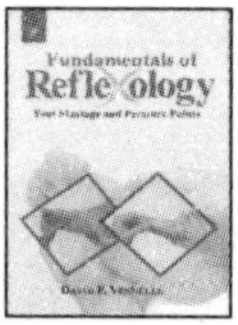

FUNDAMENTALS OF REFLEXOLOGY

Foot Massage and Pressure Points

David F. Vennells

ISBN: 81-7822-095-4

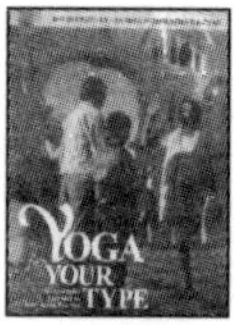

YOGA FOR YOUR TYPE

An Ayurvedic Approach to Your Asana Practice

Dr. David Frawley
Sandra Summerfield Kozak

ISBN: 81-7822-111-x

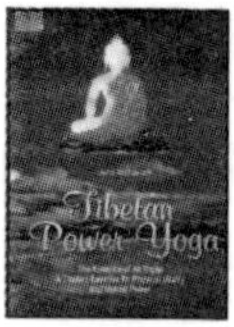

TIBETAN POWER YOGA

The Essence of All Yogas: A Tibetan Exercise for Physical Vitality and Mental Power

Jutta Mattausch

ISBN: 81-7822-006-7

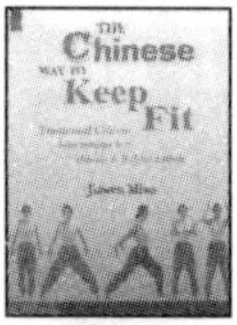

THE CHINESE WAY TO KEEP FIT

Information and Exercises

Jiawen Miao

ISBN: 81-7822-124-1

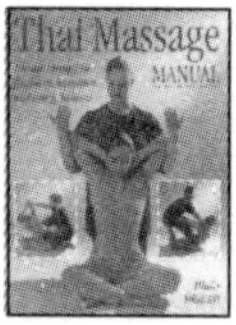

THAI MASSAGE MANUAL

A Step-by-Step Guide to Traditional Healing Techniques

Maria Mercati

ISBN: 81-7822-222-1

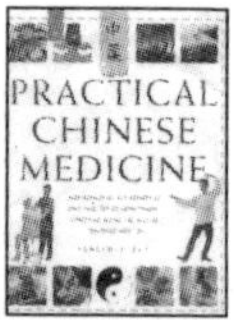

PRACTICAL CHINESE MEDICINE

Understanding the Principles and Practice of Traditional Chinese Medicine and Making them Work for You

Penelope Ody

ISBN: 81-7822-123-3